MALNUTRITION AND BRAIN DEVELOPMENT

Malnutrition and Brain Development

MYRON WINICK, M.D.

R. R. Williams Professor of Nutrition
Professor of Pediatrics
Director, Institute of Human Nutrition
Columbia University College of Physicians and Surgeons

New York
Oxford University Press
London   1976   Toronto

PREFACE

During the past two decades, evidence has accumulated from a number of sources suggesting that malnutrition during early life can impair the biochemical and functional development of the brain. Perhaps more ominously, this evidence also suggests that part if not all of the impairment may be permanent. In this book, I have tried to select the most important animal and human studies, to evaluate them, and to develop an overall picture of the consequences of early malnutrition on brain structure and function.

Chapter I is an overview of the problem of malnutrition during the growing period. It documents not only the severity and the extent of the problem but also presents the clinical and epidemiologic evidence which has focused our attention on the developing brain. Childhood malnutrition is presented as one manifestation of a generally deprived environment, produced by complex social, economic, and cultural forces, all affecting human development.

Not only are the most severe forms of childhood malnutrition—marasmus and kwashiorkor—described, but the thesis is developed that malnutrition may affect the young child in varying degrees and that millions of children suffer from subclinical forms of the disease. Evidence of this has been collected by studying the incidence of growth failure, a universal finding among these children. It was this finding of retarded growth that first suggested that mental function might be impaired.

Chapter II considers normal brain growth in more detail. Certain aspects of structural and biochemical development of the brain which have been shown to be affected by early malnutrition are described. These include: cellular growth, myelination, carbohydrate and amino acid metabolism and transport, and protein and nucleic acid synthesis and degradation. A framework is thus laid for examining the consequences of malnutrition on brain development.

Chapter III considers in detail the effects of postnatal malnutrition on the normal cellular and biochemical processes discussed in the preceding chapter. The concept of a series of critical periods during brain development, when severe malnutrition will have maximum impact, is developed here. For example, only during hyperplastic growth is brain cell number altered by malnutrition and only during the phase of rapid myelination is the deposition of myelin curtailed. Since these critical periods do not show flexible scheduling, not only is the brain particularly vulnerable during early development but deficits induced by malnutrition at this time cannot be made up later. Thus, a reduction in brain cell number due to curtailment of the rate of cell division by early malnutrition will not be corrected by providing adequate nutrition after the normal period for brain cell division has passed. It is from this kind of reasoning that the hypothesis of permanent structural and biochemical changes induced by early malnutrition has developed. Chapter III also reviews what is currently known about the mechanisms by which malnutrition exerts these effects.

Since the most rapid biochemical and structural changes occur during prenatal brain growth, Chapter IV explores the relation between prenatal malnutrition and subsequent growth of the brain. The concept of "prenatal malnutrition" is discussed and the thesis is developed that the malnourished, poorly growing fetus may have reached that state by a number of different routes. Fetal malnutrition, then, is not a single entity but may exist in a number of forms, each different in its clinical manifestations and in its ultimate prognosis. Two types are discussed; one caused by placental vascular insufficiency and resulting in asymmetrical growth failure with a small body and a relatively large head; the other caused by maternal protein deficiency and resulting in a symmetrically growth retarded fetus. In the second case, brain size is reduced in proportion to the reduction in the size of other organs.

In this chapter, the myth of the fetus as the perfect parasite is exposed. Evidence is reviewed which demonstrates that during particular periods of gestation, the fetus is particularly vulnerable to malnutrition and that deficiencies in the maternal diet can induce impaired fetal growth.

The last chapter deals with the effects of early malnutrition on functional development of the brain. It is divided into two parts, one dealing with animal experiments and the other with human investigations.

The animal experiments document the fact that malnutrition during gestation or lactation results in behavioral changes which persist for the remainder of the animal's life. The meaning of these changes, however, is difficult to interpret and to apply to man. The best we can say is that these animals are more "emotional" and more "irritable" than normal. One interesting finding is that animals malnourished early in life when concomitantly exposed to "environmental enrichment" do not develop the behavioral abnormalities otherwise observed. This has raised the possibility that the functional effects of prenatal and postnatal malnutrition are reversible.

The human studies document the fact that children who suffer malnutrition in infancy develop poorly and are retarded in their ability to perform certain tests of intellectual function. The main problem with these studies is the complex environment in which malnutrition occurs, as described in Chapter I. This environment is one which breeds poor development, but it has not been possible to isolate malnutrition from other deprivations as the cause of intellectual deficit. In our present state of knowledge, it remains a prime suspect. The improved results attained by introducing programs of adequate early nutrition suggest that it is an important factor in retarded cognitive development.

This book, then, focuses on the effects of malnutrition on the developing brain. It brings together much evidence that early malnutrition produces structural and behavioral changes. It explores the mechanisms by which some of these changes may be induced and looks into the possibility that they can be reversed. Though all the answers are not yet in, certainly we know enough not only to design critical studies to provide the missing information but also to begin to develop national programs to protect millions of young children and unborn fetuses from man's earliest scourge—inadequate nutrition.

ACKNOWLEDGMENTS

I wish to express my gratitude to the scientists with whom I have had the privilege of working and whom are responsible for much of the data reported, particularly Dr. Jo Anne Brasel and Dr. Pedro Rosso. In addition, I would like to thank those who helped in the preparation of the manuscript—Miss Marion Blanchard who assembled all the figures, prepared the bibliography and typed and retyped much of the copy; Mr. Jeffrey House whose editorial advice and assistance were invaluable; my wife, Elaine, who edited the rougher versions and corrected the proofs; and Mr. Jaime Rozovski who helped in the preparation of the index.

New York, N.Y.   M.W.
July 1975

FIGURE ACKNOWLEDGMENTS

1–5   Varea Teran, J. Study in school age children. In: Nutricion y Desarrollo en Los Andes Ecuatorianos. Eds. Varea Teran, M., and Varea Teran, J. Quito, Ecuador, Investigaciones Medico Sociales Ecuatorianas, 1974, pp. 235–338.

1–6   Winick, M. and Rosso, P. Head circumference and cellular growth of the brain in normal and marasmic children. J. Pediat. 74:774–778, 1969.

2–1   Winick, M.: Fetal malnutrition and growth processes. Hospital Practice, May, 1970, pp. 33–41.

2–2   Winick, M. and Noble, A.: Quantitative changes in DNA, RNA and protein during prenatal and postnatal growth in the rat. Devel. Biol. 12:451–466, 1965.

2–3   Winick, M.: The effect of nutrition on cellular growth. In: Symposia of the Swedish Nutrition Foundation VII, Nutrition in Preschool Age, Ed., Blix, G. Uppsala, Almqvist and Wiksell, 1969, pp. 30–38.

2–4   Winick, M.: Nutrition and nerve cell growth. Fed. Proc. 29:1510–1515, 1970.

2–5   Dobbing, J. and Sands, J.: Timing of neuroblast multiplication in developing human brain. Adapted from Archives of Diseases in Childhood, Vol. 48, 1973, pp. 757–767.

2–6   Winick, M. and Rosso, P.: Malnutrition and cellular growth in the brain. Proc. Eighth Int'l. Cong. on Nutrition. Excerpta Medica Int'l. Cong. Series No. 213, 1970, pp. 531–538.

2–8   Winick, M.: Nutrition and nerve cell growth. Fed. Proc. 29:1510–1515, 1970.

3–1   Winick, M.: Fetal malnutrition and growth processes. Hospital Practice, May 1970, pp. 33–41.

3–2   Winick, M.: Nutrition and nerve cell growth. Fed. Proc. 29:1510–1515, 1970.

3–3   Platt, B. S.: Proteins in nutrition. Proc. Roy. Soc. B. 156:337–344, 1962.

3–4   Winick, M.: Nutrition and nerve cell growth. Fed. Proc. 29:1510–1515, 1970.

3–5   Muzzo, S. J., Beas, F., Brasel, J. A. and Gardner, L. I.: The effects of hormones and malnutrition on mitochondrial oxygen consumption and DNA synthesis in rat brain. In: Endocrine Aspects of Malnutrition. Kroc Foundation Symposia, No. 1. Eds., Gardner, L. I. and Amacher, P. Santa Ynez, Calif., Kroc Foundation, 1973, pp. 191–204.

3–6   Brasel, J. A., Jasper, H. G., and Winick M.: Influence of hormones on cell growth. In: Dietary Lipids and postnatal development. Eds., Galli,

xi

C., Jacini, G. and Pecile, A. New York, Raven Press, 1973, pp. 165–180.

3–7   Brasel, J. A. Cellular changes in intrauterine malnutrition. Chapter in: Current Concepts in Nutrition, Vol. 2, Nutrition and Fetal Development. Ed., Winick, M. New York, John Wiley and Sons, 1974, pp. 13–25.

3–8   Brasel, J. A., Jasper, H. G. and Winick, M.: Influence of hormones on cell growth. In: Dietary Lipids and Postnatal Development. Eds., Galli, C., Jacini, G. and Pecile, A. New York, Raven Press, 1973, pp. 165–180.

3–9   Brasel, J. A. and Winick, M.: Maternal nutrition and prenatal growth. Arch. Dis. Child. 47:479–485, 1972.

3–10 Jasper, H. G. and Brasel, J. A. Rat liver DNA synthesis during the "catch-up" growth of nutritional rehabilitation. J. Nutr. 104:405–414, 1974.

3–11 Winick, M. and Rosso, P.: Nutritional effects on brain DNA and proteins. In: Dietary Lipids and Postnatal Development. Eds., Galli, C., Jacini, G. and Pecile, A. New York, Raven Press, 1973, pp. 181–189.

3–12 Rosso, P. and Winick, M.: Effects of early undernutrition and subsequent refeeding on alkaline ribonuclease activity of rat cerebrum and liver. J. Nutr. (In press, 1975)

3–13 Brasel, J. A.: Cellular changes in intrauterine malnutrition. Chapter in: Current Concepts in Nutrition, Vol. 2, Nutrition and Fetal Development. Ed., Winick, M. New York, John Wiley & Sons, 1974, pp. 13–25.

3–14 Winick, M. and Rosso, P.: The effect of severe early malnutrition on cellular growth of the brain. Pediat. Res. 3:181–184, 1969.

3–15 Rosso, P., Hormazábal, J. and Winick, M.: Changes in brain weight, cholesterol, phospholipid and DNA content in marasmic children. Amer. J. Cl. Nutr. 23:1275–1279, 1970.

3–16 Rosso, P., Hormazábal, J. and Winick, M.: Changes in brain weight, cholesterol, phospholipid and DNA content in marasmic children. Amer. J. Cl. Nutr. 23:1275–1279, 1970.

3–17 Winick, M., Rosso, P. and Waterlow, J.: Cellular growth of cerebrum, cerebellum and brain stem in normal and marasmic children. Exp. Neurol. 26:393–400, 1970.

4–1   Winick, M. and Nobel, A.: Quantitative changes in ribonuclease acid and protein during normal growth of rat placenta. Nature 212:34–35, 1966.

4–2   Winick, M. and Nobel, A.: Quantitative changes in ribonuclease acid and protein during normal growth of rat placenta. Nature 212:34–35, 1966.

4–3   Rosso, P.: Transfer of nutrients across the placenta during normal gestation in the rat. Amer. J. Obstet. Gynec. (In press, 1975)

4–4   Winick, M., Coscia, A. and Nobel, A.: Cellular growth in human placenta. I. Normal placental growth. Pediat. 39:248–251, 1967.

4–5 Winick, M., Coscia, A. and Nobel, A.: Cellular growth in human placenta. I. Normal placental growth. Pediat. 39:248–251, 1967.

4–6 Minkowski, A., Roux, J., Tordet-Caridroit, C.: Pathophysiologic changes in intrauterine malnutrition. Chapter in: Current Concepts in Nutrition, Vol. 2, Nutrition and Fetal Development. Ed., Winick, M. New York, John Wiley and Sons, 1974, pp. 45–78.

4–7 Winick, M. Nutrition and nerve cell growth. Fed. Proc. 29:1510–1515, 1970.

4–8 Winick, M. Nutrition and nerve cell growth. Fed. Proc. 29:1510–1515, 1970.

4–9 Winick, M. Fetal malnutrition. Cl. Obstet. Gynec. 13:526–541, 1970.

4–10 Winick, M.: Nutrition and nerve cell growth. Fed. Proc. 29:1510–1515, 1970.

4–11 Velasco, E. G., Brasel, J. A., Sigulem, D. M., Rosso, P. and Winick, M. Effects of vascular insufficiency on placental ribonuclease activity in the rat. J. Nutr. 103:213–217, 1973.

4–14 Velasco, E. G. and Brasel, J. A.: DNA polymerase activity in normal and malnourished rat placentas. J. Pediat. 86:274–279, 1975.

4–16 Velasco, E. G., Rosso, P., Brasel, J. A. and Winick, M.: Activity of alkaline RNase in placentas of malnourished women. Amer. J. Obstet. Gynec. (In press, 1975)

4–19 Sigulem, D. M., Brasel, J. A., Velasco, E. G., Rosso, P., and Winick, M.: Plasma and urine ribonuclease as a measure of nutritional status in children. Amer. J. Cl. Nutr. 26:793–797, 1973.

5–1 Zimmermann, R. R., Geist, C. R., Strobel, D. A. and Cleveland, T. J.: Attention deficiencies in malnourished monkeys in Symposia of the Swedish Nutrition Foundation XII, Early Malnutrition and Mental Development. Eds., Cravioto, J., Hambraeus, L. and Vahlquist, B. Uppsala, Almqvist and Wiksell, 1974, pp. 115–126.

CONTENTS

MALNUTRITION AND BRAIN DEVELOPMENT

Chapter 1 **CLINICAL MALNUTRITION**

ADULT MALNUTRITION

In the adult, severe malnutrition usually leads to marked emaciation, disappearance of adipose tissue and muscle wasting to such a degree that the individual may look almost like a skeleton covered with skin. The sunken appearance of the eyes and cheeks and the protuberance of the knees and elbows are characteristics with which we have become familiar from pictures of victims of either naturally occurring or man-made starvation.

Severe famine, however, sometimes afflicts its victims differently—they become "water-logged." In adults, this type of malnutrition is called "hunger edema."[1] Why some people react to starvation in this way is not known. The edema starts insidiously first at the feet and gradually spreads upward. In very advanced cases, edema is so massive that fluid seeps out through cracks in the skin over the feet and ankles. Fluid is also present in the abdominal cavity (ascites), giving these patients a bloated, swollen appearance which contrasts sharply with the withered appearance of most victims of starvation.

Hunger edema in adults is extremely rare, occurring only in severe famines; however, it has certain features in common with kwashiorkor, which is seen in children and is much more common.

Regardless of the type of physical manifestations produced in adults suffering from severe malnutrition, a number of characteristic mental changes have been described. During the early stages of a famine, the victims' remaining energies and ingenuity are concentrated on the seeking of food. As the famine progresses, there is an extreme narrowing of interests so that food is the sole focus of thoughts and activities. Even in the most conservative societies the range of items eaten widens. Euro-

3

pean prisoners of war in Japanese camps consumed rubber tree seeds, pine needle tea, melon and pumpkin rinds, and grass and leaf extract.[2] In famines occurring in the past throughout the world anything potentially edible has been eaten. Cultural and social inhibitions disappear and men often turn against each other in competition for remaining food.

As terrible as these physical and behavioral changes have been, they are reversed if the nutritional deprivation is relieved. That is the case, at least, in adults. It may not be so in children and many reports have documented that children are especially vulnerable to the effects of severe undernutrition. Take, for example, this eyewitness account of the Irish potato famine: "Frightful and fearful is the havoc around me—the aged and the young—almost without exception swollen and ripening for the grave."[3] Petrides reported a high rate of "hunger edema" in young children in Athens during the second world war; 60% of the children were between the ages of 1 and 3.[4] Lowenstein described an "epidemic" of protein calorie malnutrition in young children who were refugees in Kasai, Congo, in 1962.[5]

Many reports have stressed the vulnerability to nutritional deprivation of children, especially toddlers, old people, sick people, and most recently pregnant and lactating women. Yet until recently little attention has been given to the possibility that malnutrition in children might be qualitatively different from malnutrition in the adult. It was assumed not only that the affliction was essentially the same but also, naturally enough, that any physical and behavioral abnormalities in children were reversible with rehabilitation.

SEVERE MALNUTRITION IN CHILDREN

Severe malnutrition in children has been traditionally classified as either infantile marasmus or kwashiorkor. Clinically, marasmus is severe emaciation in a young child, usually under the age of two. It is caused by a very low intake of both calories and protein and results in extreme wasting of the tissues of the body. The child fails to grow and therefore appears very small for his age. In this form of childhood malnutrition body homeostasis is maintained and the biochemical changes in the blood often associated with malnutrition may not appear.

Kwashiorkor is caused by a reduced protein intake while carbohydrate intake remains relatively normal. It occurs almost always in the second or third year of life when a child is weaned from the breast. It is characterized by a breakdown in body homeostasis which is manifested clinically by edema, skin lesions, hair changes, and abnormally low serum albumin levels. Although this disease, as classically described, differs considerably from marasmus, there is one striking similarity—children with kwashiorkor are also markedly retarded in growth.

Marasmus

A particularly good description of marasmus was given by Digby in 1878: "The head looked unnaturally large by contrast with the emaciated trunk, the shoulder blades projecting as if they had been inserted by mistake in too small a carcass, the arms and legs shrivelled to the size of their bones, except at the knees which are swollen."[6] This severe emaciation is the hallmark of nutritional marasmus (Fig. 1-1). Generally ascribed to a marked reduction in the intake of both calories and protein, marasmus is usually seen in young infants either weaned very early or never breast fed. The most striking feature of this disease in the young infant is growth failure. The child simply ceases to grow. Why this happens is still not known.

Another striking feature of nutritional marasmus is the apathy and hyper-irritability almost universally seen in these children. Lying in bed, they are relatively unresponsive to their environment but have periods of marked irritability, especially when moved or handled by attending personnel. These behavioral changes indicate that central nervous system dysfunction is a prominent part of the syndrome of infantile marasmus; they are not unlike the behavioral abnormalities seen in adults who have suffered severe starvation.

Another characteristic of marasmus, both in infants and in older children, is its rather gradual onset and relentless progressiveness. The more profound the calorie deprivation and the longer its duration, the worse its consequences, at least in terms of conventional clinical measurements. With mild calorie deprivation the children simply appear lean. Mid-upper-arm circumference, thigh circumference, and chest circumference do not increase at their normally expected rate. Skin fold thickness, which indicates the amount of subcutaneous fat, is decreased. Though rather slim, children appear normal. Because height is also diminished, they often seem much younger than their chronological age. Even mild calorie deprivation in a young child will impair growth. This is a qualitative dif-

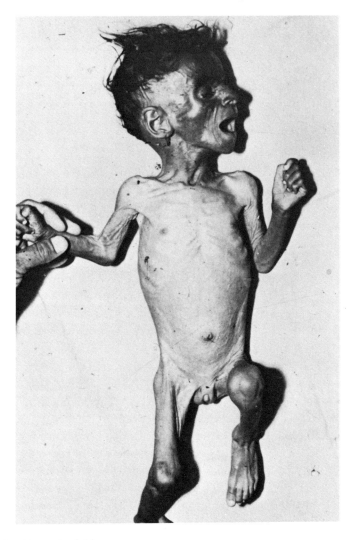

Fig. 1.1. Marasmic child

ference from calorie deprivation in the adult. The adult has passed his growing years; he has presumably reached his ultimate height and no amount of undernutrition, regardless of its type, severity, or duration, will alter his height. While this may seem apparent, it cannot be overemphasized that growth failure is the basic difference between malnutrition in children and adults.

In contrast to kwashiorkor, biochemical signs are relatively normal in patients with marasmus. Children have normal serum proteins and may not even manifest anemia.

The symptoms of marasmus disappear if treatment is successful, but the effects of growth failure in children may be permanent. All of the organs studied in marasmic children fail to reach their expected weights. The brain has been reported to be small in children who died of severe infantile marasmus in Africa,[7] in South America,[8] in Asia,[9] and in the United States.[10]

If growth stunting in children who suffer from nutritional marasmus persists throughout life this raises many questions: How many stunted adults are small because of inadequate nutrition in infancy? What is the significance, if any, of being small? Is there any compensating mechanism for reduction in brain growth early in life? What are the functional implications of a permanently stunted brain?

Kwashiorkor

Kwashiorkor commonly affects weanling children in many parts of the world. It is characterized by edema, skin and hair changes, apathy, and growth failure (Fig. 1-2). The metabolic changes caused by kwashiorkor are quite different from those of marasmus. In the chronic protein deficiency leading to kwashiorkor there are biochemical alterations which reflect difficulties in the maintenance of homeostasis. During simple starvation, the rapid breakdown of tissues not only supplies energy for essential requirements but also supplies metabolites for the synthesis of certain important compounds necessary for maintaining the body's functions. The concentrations of free amino acids in the serum, for example, are essentially normal and serum albumin concentration is maintained. By contrast, in children who have frank kwashiorkor or who consume low-protein high-carbohydrate diets, tissue catabolism is reduced since sufficient energy is available from the carbohydrate in the diet. Thus there is depletion of essential amino acids and reduced synthesis of certain proteins such as serum albumin.

Despite these general differences between marasmus and kwashiorkor (and certain specific differences which we will describe), the earliest change in both these conditions is the same—failure to grow at the normal rate. In kwashiorkor, metabolic processes associated with growth breakdown. For example, the synthesis of collagen for connective tissue, bone,

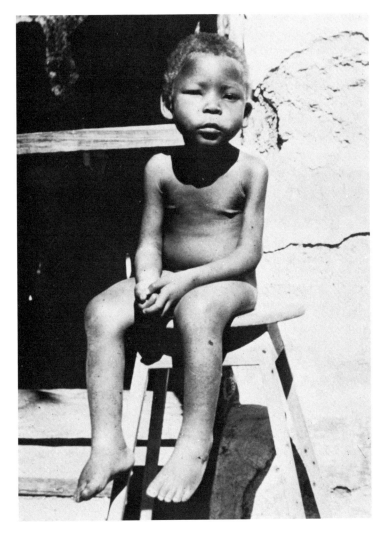

Fig. 1.2. Child with kwashiorkor

and skin is markedly impaired. This impairment is reflected by the reduced excretion of hydroxyproline-containing peptides in the urine of
these children. In addition, the low intake of protein at a time when
requirements for protein are high results in a reduction in the excretion
of urea and in the ratio of urea to creatinine in the urine. These metabolic
changes can be interpreted as an attempt by the body to conserve pro-

tein. This concept is strengthened by the observation that the activity of certain cellular enzymes associated with protein synthesis increases while that of enzymes involved in urea production decreases. Thus both kwashiorkor and marasmus elicit a similar protein-conserving reaction.

Other biochemical alterations, however, appear to be specific for kwashiorkor. Certain serum amino acids, particularly valine, are normally present in concentrations varying between 200 and 399 μM/L. In a child living on low-protein, relatively high carbohydrate intake, valine concentration drops to 90 to 150 μM/L. The intake in protein is apparently inadequate to meet the needs of growth. But in addition, the reduced tissue breakdown, especially of muscle, does not supply enough amino acids to replenish the amino acid pool. The reason for this lack of tissue breakdown is unclear but it may be related to the relatively high carbohydrate content of the diet, which increases circulating insulin, a hormone known to inhibit tissue breakdown.[11]

Hair changes are a characteristic feature of kwashiorkor and may be one of the earliest signs of disease. Changes appear first around the temples where the hair becomes sparse and less pigmented. In some cases, the child's hair will become blond (Fig. 1-3). In other cases zones of depigmentation may alternate with zones of normal-appearing hair. The depigmentated blond areas presumably reflect periods of severe protein deprivation. In addition, a number of morphologic changes in the hair fibers and roots seem to be specific for kwashiorkor.[12] The basis for all these hair changes is still unknown. As they appear early in the course of the disease, the hair changes may reflect the body's attempt to conserve protein and reduce nitrogen loss by depriving a tissue whose function is relatively unimportant.

As a child develops frank kwashiorkor, his face becomes rounded. This "moon face" may be barely noticeable at first, but as the disease progresses there is no mistaking its presence. Its exact pathogenesis is not clear but seems to involve a tendency to accumulate subcutaneous fat and extracellular water. The accumulation of extracellular water (edema) is the most dramatic sign of kwashiorkor. In this disease edema is pitting in nature and in a toddler usually appears first in the lower extremities and then progresses upward over the entire body (Fig. 1-4). Though the metabolic causes of edema are complex and still not entirely understood, it is almost invariably associated with a reduced serum albumin concentration. There is evidence that the control of sodium reabsorption is impaired, leading to a retention of sodium and consequently of

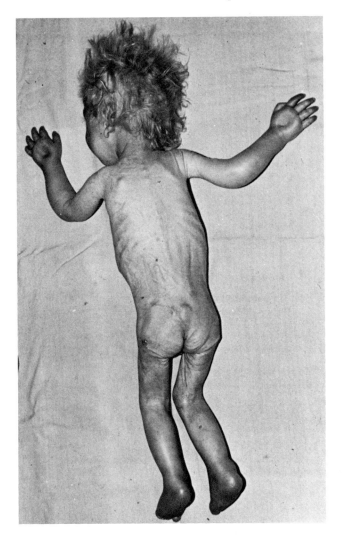

Fig. 1.3.   Hair changes in kwashiorkor

water. The appearance of edema early in the disease is often intermittent, waxing and waning when the serum albumin concentration falls to around 3 gms %. As the albumin level falls to 2.5 gms %, edema tends to persist. Thus, serum albumin values below 3 gms % are a warning sign of kwashiorkor.

There has been a great deal of study and speculation concerning the

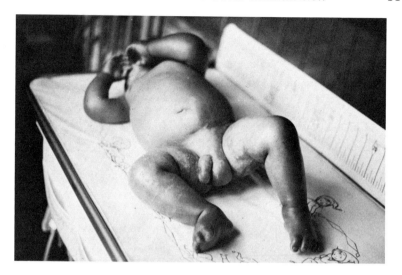

Fig. 1.4. Edema of the legs in kwashiorkor

cause of the low serum albumin values in kwashiorkor. Even under moderate to severe conditions of malnutrition the ability to synthesize proteins is relatively well maintained. For some reason, however, albumin synthesis is reduced. It has been postulated that too little substrate is available at the site of albumin synthesis in liver tissue and that this may be due in part to the excess of available carbohydrate which diverts amino acids to muscle rather than liver cells. In the normal child this "protein-sparing" action of carbohydrate is beneficial; however, in the child suffering from primary deficiency it may be detrimental.[11] Regardless of the mechanism by which it is produced, low circulating albumin concentration is clearly the main biochemical feature of kwashiorkor.

Another feature of this type of undernutrition is a tendency to accumulate fat in the liver. Again, the cause is unclear, but it has been speculated that there may be a lack of the lipoprotein carrier necessary for the transport of fat from the liver once it has been synthesized.[13]

In contrast to marasmus, then, the development of kwashiorkor is characterized by a number of metabolic derangements and major difficulties in the maintenance of homeostasis. Among these abnormalities are extracellular edema, low serum albumin, distorted serum aminogram, and fat accumulation in the liver. As we have seen, there are also certain similarities between both extreme types of malnutrition in children. These include a failure to grow properly and certain behavioral abnormalities, and both may have permanent effects.

Protein calorie malnutrition

Since anorexia is often an important part of kwashiorkor, the effects of starvation may also be evident. Thus we have a child who as a consequence of kwashiorkor develops superimposed marasmus. This has led to the concept of a spectrum with kwashiorkor at one end, marasmus at the other, and marasmic-kwashiorkor in the middle. The child with marasmic-kwashiorkor suffers varying degrees of emaciation, edema, low serum albumin, etc. Since a large number of malnourished children fall into this group some people have used the term "protein calorie malnutrition" (PCM) to describe all forms of childhood malnutrition.

It has also been recognized that despite the differences between malnutrition in children and in adults there may be a continuum between the childhood and adult forms of the disease. Marasmus in the infant does resemble starvation in the adult and the recent experience in eastern Nigeria (Biafra) after the civil war has demonstrated similarities between kwashiorkor in children and hunger edema in adults.[14] Many cases of ascites associated with protein-calorie malnutrition were observed there.[14] One of the main differences between childhood kwashiorkor and adult hunger edema was thought to be the lack of ascites in the former and its universal presence in the latter, yet ascites was present most often in the children who had kwashiorkor. Data on 100 children under 15 years of age showed ascites associated with edema and quite often with features of kwashiorkor, such as skin and hair changes. All of these patients had low levels of serum albumin when investigated, and perhaps more significantly the ascites subsided with the generalized edema in 1 to 5 weeks on a high-protein diet alone.

Another manifestation of protein-calorie malnutrition in children, hypoglycemia, bears mentioning both because in Biafra it was the commonest cause of death from nutritional deprivation, especially in severe cases of marasmus, and because it is a common manifestation of another type of malnutrition which we will discuss shortly—fetal malnutrition. In Biafran children episodes of hypoglycemia occurred most frequently in the early hours of the morning because of the long fast between dinner and breakfast. The onset of weakness, drowsiness, and coma was sudden. The children would begin gasping for breath and sometimes muscle twitching and generalized convulsions would follow. Unless treatment was prompt, death occurred in 5 to 15 minutes. Yet the process was quickly reversed by the administration of hypertonic glucose solution (20-50%) and feeding every three hours around the clock prevented hypoglycemia.[14]

Other diseases accompanying malnutrition

Anemia, though not essential to the diagnosis of protein-calorie malnutrition, is present more often than not. Again drawing on the recent experience in Biafra,[14] in a group of 500 malnourished children investigated, 70% had hemoglobin counts between 4 and 9 gms %, 18% had hemoglobin levels below 4 gms %, and 3% recorded levels below 2 gms %. The causes of anemia included malaria, ancylostomiasis, deficiencies of specific nutrients such as iron or folic acid, infections, and hemoglobinopathies.

Diarrhea often accompanies malnutrition, particularly marasmus. This is a very serious complication for it aggravates malnutrition, produces dehydration, and makes therapy extremely difficult since intravenous feeding is almost always required.

Infection is an equally serious problem when associated with malnutrition in young children. The weak, wasting child is more prone to infection and, when contracted, infectious diseases are much more severe in malnourished children. Extremely high death rates from measles, for instance, have been reported in developing countries.[15] Although early students of the problem ascribed the difference in African and European death rates from measles to a more virulent measles virus, it has become plain that the difference is not in the virus but in the response to the virus by the host. Well-nourished children of elite Nigerian families do not respond very differently to an attack of measles than children in most parts of Europe and America. In contrast, malnourished children show increased morbidity and mortality, and in children who are severely malnourished the death rate from measles can be as high as 50%.[16]

The incidence of tuberculosis is increased in malnourished populations and the disease progresses much more rapidly in malnourished patients.[17] There is an increased susceptibility to gastrointestinal infections in children who are malnourished.[18] Hepatitis, Herpes Simplex, and typhus fever have all been reported to be more severe in severely undernourished children.[19]

The mechanisms by which a malnourished host is more easily infected and more disabled by bacteria or viruses are not clearly understood. Recent work in both animals and man suggests that both humoral and cellular immune reactions are affected by malnutrition. It has even been suggested that these altered immune responses may persist for long periods after amelioration of the malnutrition. There is evidence that as malnutrition becomes more severe the transmission rate of certain infections increases. The Crusaders' ranks were often decimated by famine and epidemics. Thousands died of plague and typhus during the Russian famine of 1602, and, in Italy after the thirty-year war, malnutrition in the population was associated with one of the worst outbreaks of typhus fever ever recorded.[20] The combined effects of undernutrition and epidemics of infectious diseases have perhaps been clearest in military sieges. The combination of undernutrition and pestilence reduced an army of 300,000 to 60,000 during the siege of Antioch in 1098.[20] During the siege of Danzig in 1813 the same combination resulted in more than 7000 deaths among the 36,000 defenders within a 60-day period. Thirty thousand French soldiers died of malnutrition and epidemic infectious disease during the Torgau siege in 1813. During the siege of Paris that lasted from September 1870 until February 1871, daily food rations decreased periodically. In the week before the armistice was signed, five times as many people died as would have been expected by comparison with the same week in previous years. Smallpox, typhoid fever, dysentery and diarrhea, pneumonia, and bronchitis accounted for over 40% of the 4671 deaths in that week[21]

Just as malnutrition may have permanent sequelae, so may infections. Thus, when we observe an individual "damaged" as an adult, we cannot know whether this damage was induced by previous malnutrition, by previous infection or, as is most often the case, by a combination of the two.

NUTRITION AND PHYSICAL GROWTH

So far we have described some of the effects of severe malnutrition on two vulnerable groups—infants and young children. The most striking similarity between these groups is that they are rapidly growing. Let us now examine in more detail some of the effects of undernutrition on growth.

Growth has classically been measured in terms of height and weight, and the former is the best indication of over-all body growth. It is also a relatively simple measurement to make, and much of our epidemiologic data about the effects of undernutrition on growth derives from this measurement. A child's increase in height is not a smooth progression but occurs rapidly during certain periods and more slowly during others. Growth is rapid during fetal life and early infancy, it slows down in early childhood, almost ceases before puberty, and then spurts up again until adult size is reached. Final height depends on the rate of growth during these phases and on their duration. Malnutrition during infancy and childhood reduces height before adolescence (Fig. 1-5) and, in addition, delays the onset of adolescence. The growth rate during adolescence is also curtailed and the individual will be sexually mature at a far smaller than normal size, often reaching adulthood 4 to 6 inches below average height.

Behind the smaller size of malnourished children lie larger differences in the composition of the body. Severe malnutrition may reduce lean body mass by as much as 35%. If malnutrition continues into adulthood, the amount of body fat may be less than one-third of normal.[22]

Maturity can be measured by assessing bone maturation with radio-

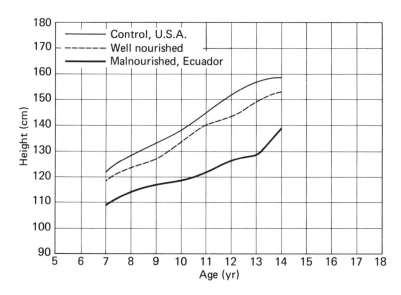

Fig. 1.5.   Height—female school children from Ecuador and the United States

graphic techniques. In severe malnutrition, there is a delay in the appearance of certain ossification centers. The delay can be very specific and therefore helpful in determining the degree of maturational arrest. For example, in Guatemala, El Salvador, and Costa Rica the delay in the appearance of the adductor sesamoid is not nearly so great as the delay in the appearance of the trapezium, the trapezoid, the navicular, and the distal ulna.[23] Thus a delay in the last four ossification centers implies moderate undernutrition. If in addition the adductor sesamoid is delayed, the undernutrition must have been severe.

Recently the time of appearance of ossification centers has been determined in a population of Navajo Indian children living on a reservation in the United States.[24] Three hundred and eleven standardized hand-wrist radiographs of 159 boys and 152 girls aged 6 months to 17 years were studied to determine skeletal maturation and bone mineralization. When compared to standards for white American children, the skeletal maturation of these children was delayed on the average 14% in boys and 30% in girls. This is equivalent to 1 year and 1½ to 2 years of growth respectively. In contrast, reduction in size was greater in boys (1.4 years) than in girls (0.5 years).

Among several other indices of body composition, the most useful have been mid-upper-arm circumference and thickness of the triceps muscle. Mid-upper-arm circumference is a simple, valuable measure of muscle mass. It correlates well with determinations of muscle mass made by more sophisticated and complicated techniques. Its use in Africa and the Caribbean has shown that total muscle mass is reduced in malnourished children.[25] This reduction has been confirmed by direct measurement of triceps muscle thickness with calipers, a slightly more difficult technique to employ under field conditions. Skin calipers have also been used to estimate total body fat. Measurement of thoracic fat fold thickness, for example, revealed a reduction in total body fat in White Mountain Apache children.[26]

The measurement most germane to our discussion is that of head circumference. Except under grossly pathologic conditions brain growth correlates with head circumference, and this correlation holds in normal and malnourished children.[27] The relation between head circumference and intelligence as measured by standard I.Q. tests adapted for various populations has also been studied. In affluent, well-nourished populations there is no correlation between head circumference and intelligence until the head circumference is reduced to such a magnitude that microcephaly is present and obvious brain pathology exists. In marked contrast, there is a high correlation between reduced head circumference and reduced intelligence in poor malnourished populations.[28]

Numerous studies have demonstrated that malnutrition, especially during gestation and the first two to three years of life, will retard the rate of increase in head circumference, and leave the older child or adult with a permanently reduced cranial volume (Fig. 1-6). This reduction in cranial circumference has been reported in almost every developing country in the world. It was the first alarming sign that permanent brain damage might result from early malnutrition. The earlier the malnutrition, the more marked is the reduction of head circumference.[29] The marasmic child, then, is much more apt to have reduced cranial circumference than the child with kwashiorkor—not because of the differences in the two disease processes but because of the younger age at which marasmus develops. From the standpoint of physical growth, and more particularly of ultimate brain growth, marasmus is a much more serious

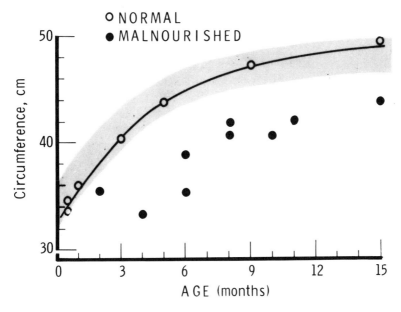

Fig. 1.6. Head circumference in normal and malnourished children

disease than kwashiorkor. In addition, moderate and even mild undernutrition very early in life may retard brain growth more than severe malnutrition later in life. Thus the time in life when malnutrition occurs is crucial to brain growth. This is an essential point because the pattern of undernutrition throughout the world is shifting in the direction of younger and younger children.

To understand this shift we must understand the entire ecology of malnutrition. Malnutrition does not occur in a vacuum but is the product of specific environments, environments which are all too common within our modern world.

THE ECOLOGY OF MALNUTRITION

The best studies of the "ecology of malnutrition" have been carried out by Cravioto and his colleagues in Guatemala and Mexico.[30, 31, 32, 33] They have pointed out that because of the intimate association between nutritional status and income levels in almost all societies, children who are at the highest risk for malnutrition will be clustered in that segment of society which is poorest and socially most deprived. This deprived group, of course, also differs from the rest of society in other respects. For example, they have poorer, more dilapidated housing, and they are more prone to follow traditional methods of child care and hold irrational concepts of health and disease. Furthermore, a broad socio-cultural change is occurring that may have serious consequences for the nutrition of children of the poor in the developing world. Especially among the urban poor of "third world" countries, marked shortening in the period of breast feeding has taken place. Throughout Africa and Latin America breast feeding is on the decline despite concerted efforts by public health officials to promote it. In Chile, breast feeding is uncommon. By the time the infant is three months old, more than 80% of Chilean mothers are no longer breast feeding.[34] A free milk program was instituted about 15 years ago and has been expanded considerably by succeeding administrations, particularly the government of Salvador Allende. Before this program began, Chile had the highest infant mortality in South America, though over-all childhood mortality was relatively low. After 12 years of wide distribution of free powdered milk, especially in urban ghettos, the infant mortality in Chile was still the highest in South America. In fact, it did not decrease significantly. Living conditions help explain the failure of the free milk program. The typical home in Santiago's slums is a one-room shack, built of stone and wood and roofed with corrugated tin. There are no sanitary facilities, no running water, no refrigeration. The cooking is done in a large garbage can converted for that purpose. Under these conditions, the mother receiving powdered milk is expected to prepare a formula in a sterile manner for her small infant. After the milk powder has been mixed with contaminated water in dirty bottles and left to stand at room temperature part of the day, this product of modern technology is likely to produce diarrhea. If the mother stops using milk powder and reverts to the mixtures of flour and water (a poor culture medium) used in the past, the diarrhea may subside but the child may become marasmic.

The moon faces and bloated bellies of kwashiorkor are becoming less familiar sights throughout the world. In Lebanon, Turkey, Peru, Iran, and other countries, recent reports indicate that marasmus is becoming the most common type of malnutrition. As in Chile, the child suffering from marasmus anywhere in the world usually belongs to a family living in a crowded town or city. Often neither parent has a secure job. A history of sudden, early weaning due to repeated pregnancy is very common. The child is bottle fed and receives a highly contaminated diet of low nutritional value, which results in repeated bouts with diarrhea. Because of the diarrhea, feeding is restricted and this further complicates the child's nutritional problems.

Figure 1-7 shows the age distribution of childhood malnutrition in Teheran hospitals in 1966. More than 50% of the children were under one year of age. Over 80% were under two years of age. Malnutrition, especially in urban areas, is becoming primarily a disorder of infants.[35]

The decline in breast feeding is probably the largest factor contributing to the development of malnutrition in very young children today. Just why this trend has gained momentum is not at all clear. City life, especially for newcomers, is full of uncertainty: job opportunities are scarce; food is expensive; living conditions are crowded and unhygienic. This environment is certainly not conducive to breast feeding. If the mother works, breast feeding is impractical. Advertising of formulas and commercial baby food tends to downgrade the value of breast feeding.

Figure 1-8 shows what has happened to breast feeding in two different communities: a section of urban Teheran and a nearby rural area. Although 80% of the mothers in the urban area started breast feeding only 40% continued for more than three months. By the end of six months

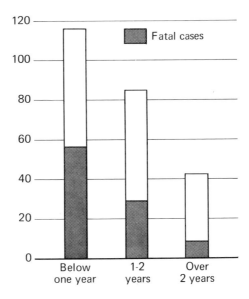

Fig. 1.7. Malnutrition by age in hospitalized children

only 20% continued to nurse and even in these women the quantity of milk was reduced, as assessed by the infants' weight gain. In the rural area, 80% of the mothers continued to breast feed successfully for at least 12 months.

Industrialization in the cities of developing countries has provoked a migration from villages by creating a demand for labor. The big city has a great attraction for rural populations, but the price they must pay is also great. Bottle feeding is just one more economic burden for an already overburdened family. In developing countries the cost of feeding a young infant with commercial baby formula can be up to 25% of a laborer's salary. Such an expense is obviously prohibitive and the result equally obvious—malnutrition of the infant.

The shifting pattern of malnutrition toward younger and younger children is a product of emerging technology in previously underdeveloped countries. It is an attempt to utilize one element of technology, artificial infant feeding, before other elements such as purified water, refrigeration, and devices for food preparation are available.

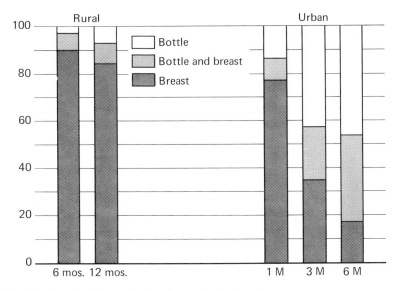

Fig. 1.8.   Length of breast feeding in rural and urban Iran

SUBCLINICAL MALNUTRITION

Discussing this shift in malnutrition to earlier age groups only in terms of the increase in frank marasmus is a little like concentrating on the tip of an iceberg. By using anthropomorphic measures like height and mid-upper-arm circumference, together with certain biochemical tests, the extent of the problem in less severely affected children can be determined. Such surveys have been performed in many countries throughout the world.[36]

In the developing world the death rate from malnutrition is about 5 to 10 per thousand children, but those who live to suffer the effects of malnutrition are far more numerous. In Uganda it has been estimated that 5000 to 7000 children aged 1 to 5 die of malnutrition annually. In the same country, clinical malnutrition (that is, frank symptoms and signs of nutritional disorder) is estimated to exist in 1-2% of all children. Thus, at any given time 10,000 to 20,000 children in Uganda are grossly malnourished. Similar statistics are available for underdeveloped countries throughout the world. They indicate that even by the most conservative estimates millions of children in the world today show objective signs of severe malnutrition.

As we have seen, one standard measure of malnutrition in early life is subsequent height. Together with biochemical determinations of certain nutrients in the blood this measurement has been used in surveys conducted throughout the world in an attempt to document the incidence of childhood malnutrition. These studies require proper standards of comparison and relative assurance of the child's age and they are not always easy to obtain in developing countries. It would be much less troublesome in a country like the United States with sophisticated recording systems, but until five years ago we had not conducted such a survey in the United States.

In a survey based on anthropometry alone a minimum of 30% of the entire childhood population of Uganda was retarded in growth when compared to a local standard for height. This comes to 336,000 children in this single African country. In a more recent study in the same country, where biochemical as well as anthropomorphic data were gathered, it was found that about 50% of the children up to 4 years old in three districts of Uganda showed either biochemical signs of protein imbalance or growth retardation, or both. On a nationwide basis this would be more than half a million children. Findings such as these are unfortunately consistent in many developing countries throughout the world. They indicate that perhaps 300 million people alive today have suffered some degree of malnutrition early in life.

MALNUTRITION IN THE UNITED STATES

We are now beginning to learn that malnutrition, usually considered a problem of underdevelopment, exists in many parts of the United States.

If we examine the living conditions of the American Indians, it becomes clear that there is an "underdeveloped society" within our own country.[37] Conditions of life among the Navajo Indians in Arizona differ very little from those of rural populations in parts of Latin America, Africa, and Asia. A few demographic and socioeconomic facts should serve to illustrate this similarity. About 44% of the American Indian population live in one-room houses, the traditional hogans. Thirty-five per cent of the population live in dwellings with no sanitary facilities. Few families have piped water or wells adjacent to their homes. Twenty-eight per cent of the men and 43% of the women have no schooling; nearly 50% of adults have less than four years of schooling. Thirty-six per cent of the men work less than full time on a year-round basis.

Substandard housing, poor sanitation, inadequate water supply, unemployment, lack of education—the same circumstances that Cravioto described in Guatemala and Mexico—breed malnutrition in American Indians.[37] The purchasing power for adequate nutrition is simply not there. This could actually be determined in the Navajo population by identifying per capita food expenditures, which decreased as family size increased. Households of three, four, and five members reported weekly per capita food purchases at a rate of $7.00, $5.27, and $4.54, respectively. When family size increased to nine or more persons, weekly per capita food expenditures fell to $2.99. Thus, in 1969, when these findings were reported, the average Navajo family was spending between forty cents and a dollar a day per person for food. Given the cost of living in this country, this amount of money is obviously unlikely to provide enough food for a proper diet.

The majority of infants were bottle fed. Breast feeding with or without supplementation was practiced by only about one-third of the mothers. The use of milk or a milk-based formula was highest with children under 3; over half the children between 3 and 6 consumed almost no milk. Many Navajo mothers thought milk caused diarrhea and hence did not give it to their infants.

Examination of the Navajo children revealed clear-cut manifestations of malnutrition. Signs of riboflavin deficiency, iodine deficiency, dental caries, and fluorosis of the teeth were very common. Laboratory examinations revealed anemia in 17% of the children and low serum iron levels in 23%. Five per cent of the entire population, mostly in the older age groups, had low vitamin C levels. Eleven per cent of the males and 14% of the females had levels of serum proteins below those considered acceptable by the National Nutrition Survey.

Perhaps most striking were the anthropomorphic findings. Nearly 50% of children under 4 years of age fell below the tenth percentile for weight. Sixty-eight per cent of infants under three had head circumferences below the tenth percentile of the Boston growth standard.

In a similar survey, it was found that Apache children 1 to 6 years of age living on an Indian reservation in Arizona had mean intakes of calories, calcium, vitamin A, vitamin C, and vitamin B12 substantially below those that were considered sufficient for optimal health. The protein in their diets was sufficient in quantity but poor in quality and in many instances it may have been utilized to meet energy needs because calorie intake was low. Increase in height was significantly retarded. Most of these Apache children were ingesting insufficient iron to meet current needs or to create adequate stores.

Congressional hearings early in 1967 had first dramatized the probability that serious hunger and malnutrition existed in the United States. Later that year, Congress directed the Department of Health, Education and Welfare to determine the scope of malnutrition and related health problems in this country. Because no body of evidence existed, it was decided to conduct a nutritional survey to carry out this directive.[38] Constraints of time and money limited the survey to ten states: Washington, California, Texas, Louisiana, South Carolina, Kentucky, West Virginia, Michigan, Massachusetts, and New York (including a separate survey of New York City). The choice also reflected the states' supply of trained manpower and other available resources, and *whether or not they wished to be surveyed*. Most of the people surveyed were poor and they came from white, black, and Spanish American populations in that order.

The survey indicated that many of these people were malnourished or at high risk of developing nutritional problems. However, malnutrition in different segments of the population surveyed varied in severity and in regard to the nutrients involved. One clear example of this variation was the high prevalence of vitamin A deficits among Mexican Americans in states with a low average income, compared with the absence of vitamin A problems among Puerto Ricans in states with a high average income such as New York.

Because the type and degree of malnutrition vary from one locality to another, generalizations tend to be misleading. In this survey, however, evidence of malnutrition was found most commonly among blacks, less often among Spanish Americans, and least among white persons. Generally, evidence of malnutrition increased as income level decreased. Among the various age groups surveyed, poor nutritional status was most common in adolescents between the ages of 10 and 16 years, and boys showed more evidence of malnutrition than girls. Iron deficiency was common within the entire population surveyed and surprisingly was often present in adolescent and adult males. Protein intake was marginal in many pregnant and lactating women and vitamin A levels were low, especially among Spanish Americans.

Thus within the past five years it has become quite clear that malnutrition, a disease thought alien to the United States, is a significant problem in a large segment of our population.

PRENATAL UNDERNUTRITION

In addition to the clear evidence that infants are especially vulnerable to the effects of malnutrition, it is now being recognized that maternal malnutrition during pregnancy may result in inadequate growth of the fetus. Moreover, after childbirth the mother's ability to lactate properly may be impaired. With mild nutritional deprivation, lactation is usually only slightly affected so that breast-fed babies have a margin of safety. In Athens during World War II, for instance, Petrides found no "hunger edema" in infants less than six months of age.[4] He believed that babies either received no breast milk and died, or received a "basal" amount of breast milk and survived. This protective effect of breast feeding was noted in Rotterdam toward the end of World War II,[39] in the Congo in the early 1960's[5] and during the siege of Leningrad,[40] where Antonov observed that "as long as the mammary gland received sufficient physical stimulation, milk continued to be secreted, although the quantity might be reduced and the length of lactation shortened."

The incidence of breast feeding is reported to have increased during the siege of Paris in 1876, with a *decline* in infant mortality despite the rising mortalities in other age groups.[41] Similarly, in Japanese internment camps, European and American women breast fed their babies successfully for about one year.[42]

With severe chronic malnutrition of lifelong duration the situation is quite different. Lactation declines and eventually ceases. The young infant is no longer protected and marasmus and diarrheal disease begin to develop.[43]

Severe maternal malnutrition will also affect both the mother and the developing fetus during gestation. It may lead to amenorrhea and to increased rates of stillbirths.[39, 40] "Starvation amenorrhea" functions protectively by conserving menstrual blood and hence reducing the "nutritional loss."[44] In addition, marked malnutrition is associated with a decline in libido, infertility, and a consequent drop in birth rates.[45, 46]

In some ways this reduced fertility in severely undernourished women has led to a false sense of security. Little attention was given to the possibility that the fetus might not grow properly within this type of maternal environment. It was felt that if a woman was able to become pregnant, she was nourished well enough to carry the fetus to term. The concept of the fetus as a perfect parasite was prevalent in most developed countries. Obstetricians were recommending strict weight control during pregnancy. Many even felt that this period of life could be used to effect weight reduction. Even today we can read in current "diet books" of weight reduction programs which are said to be safe for pregnant women. This sense of the protection of the fetus was reinforced by the commonly held view of prematurity as a matter of birth weight only. Any newborn weighing 2500 grams or less was defined as premature. Useful as this definition was, it created the impression that all small infants were born before term. The increased incidence of small but full-term babies in women from malnourished populations was interpreted as the result of an increased rate of prematurity. Recently, however, we have begun to separate small babies into two major categories: the true premature who is the right size for his fetal age but is born too soon and the so-called small-for-dates infant who is born on time but has not grown properly *in utero* and is therefore small on delivery.

These small-for-dates infants have been further divided into two groups: those with "intrinsic" growth failure and those with "extrinsic" growth failure mediated by certain abnormalities in the fetal environment.[47] Intrinsic growth failure results from congenital malformation, inborn errors of metabolism, and other genetic diseases. It is interesting that although these infants are small, their placentas are generally of normal size. This suggests that whatever the mechanism for the growth failure, it is intrinsic to the fetus and does not involve the placenta.

At least two categories of extrinsic growth failure can be described.[48] The first, which we will arbitrarily call Type 1 growth failure, is characterized by asymmetry. The various fetal organs are affected differently. The brain is almost entirely spared, while the liver is markedly reduced in size and totally depleted in glycogen. The other type of extrinsic fetal growth failure (Type 2) is symmetrical in its effects on the various organs. Brain and liver are both reduced in size, but they are reduced to the same degree that body size is. In both these extrinsic types of growth failure, placental growth is also curtailed. A diagram of this classification is given below.

Type 1 fetal growth failure is most commonly caused by maternal vascular disease which results in a reduced blood supply to the fetus.

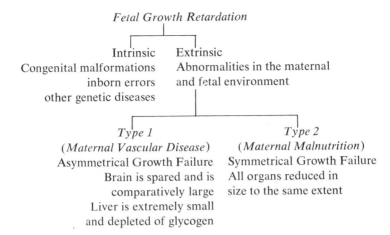

Fig. 1.9. Classification of fetal growth retardation

Type 2 fetal growth failure is most commonly associated with maternal malnutrition. Both types can be produced in experimental animals. Type 1 fetal growth failure characterizes the vast majority of small-for-dates infants in developed societies. Type 2 is the much more prevalent form in developing countries and probably within the poorer segments of our own country.

This concept that small-for-dates infants make up a large part of the group of supposedly premature infants has cast an entirely different light on the problem of maternal malnutrition. Smith's report of an increased rate of prematurity during the Dutch famine of 1944-45, for example, failed to discern that many of these babies, perhaps the vast majority, could have been small-for-dates infants subjected to severe undernutrition during gestation.[39] The over-all drop in birth weight in this previously well-nourished population was about 200 grams—a figure that is quite significant. This difference of 200 grams corresponds to the average difference in birth weight between rich and poor in the developed countries of the world. During the siege of Leningrad the effects were even more marked.[40] The average birth weight dropped about 400 grams during this period of severe nutritional deprivation.

For years we have known that birth weights were lower in developing countries than in more advanced areas of the world. We have also known that birth weights among poor people in the United States were lower than among the rich. Tentative explanations of these differences have been based on genetic factors and, more recently, on poor nutrition.

The increase in birth weight in Japan over the past two decades lends support to a nutritional explanation.[49] Although many changes in addition to improvement in nutrition have occurred in Japan during this period, certainly the genetic or racial factor has remained the same. Furthermore, it has been shown that second-generation Japanese in the United States are on the average several inches taller than their fathers.[50] This difference can be explained at least in part by the different diet consumed by the mothers during pregnancy.

Infant mortality correlates directly with low birth weight. In fact, the difference in perinatal mortality between developed and developing countries can be explained on the basis of low birth weight alone.[51] In our own country the difference in infant mortality between the poor and the wealthy almost corresponds to the difference in birth weight. If birth weights are equal, poor babies survive as well as rich babies, black babies as well as white babies.[51] If malnutrition of the mother makes a significant contribution to low birth weight, then adequate feeding during pregnancy should increase birth weight and diminish fetal mortality. As we shall soon see, improved maternal feeding does have that effect.[52]

There are two other strong epidemiologic arguments for the important role of maternal nutrition in fetal growth. The first is that birth weight correlates with increase in maternal weight.[53] Within limits, the more the mother gains during pregnancy the larger the baby. The optimal amount of weight gain has not been determined and will no doubt vary depending on the mother's previous nutritional status. At present, the committee on maternal nutrition of the National Academy of Sciences recommends a weight gain of at least 25 pounds for previously well-nourished women.[54] This is a far cry from the practices of the past when women were told to keep their weight gain to less than 10 pounds or to gain no weight at all, or actually to reduce.

The second piece of epidemiologic evidence implicating the nutritional status of the mother in fetal growth is the relation between maternal size and birth weight.[55] In affluent societies there is no correspondence between these two variables. In developing countries, however, where maternal height reflects previous nutrition, there is a direct correlation between maternal height and infant weight at birth. The smaller the mother, the smaller her infant. Several studies have indicated that this direct correlation has a nutritional rather than genetic basis.

The most compelling evidence of the direct relationship between maternal nutrition and infant birth weight comes from a study in Guate-

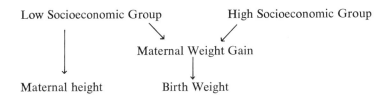

Fig. 1.10. Nutritional influences on birth weight

mala where the diet of the entire population of a poor village was supplemented with either a high caloric or a high protein drink.[52] Data accumulated so far indicate that increasing either the calories or the protein in the diet of pregnant women in the village increased birth weights by approximately 300 grams. This is theoretically enough to explain the difference in perinatal mortality between poor and rich Guatemalans. Not enough cases have yet been studied to establish whether in fact the neonatal death rate has changed as much. For this population, it seems that 20,000 extra calories delivered to the mother throughout the entire pregnancy is the amount necessary to produce a birth weight gain of about 300 grams. Moreover, it does not matter much whether these calories are provided throughout the entire 10 months of gestation or for only part of the period. What is critical is the amount (20,000 calories). Apparently the mother is somehow able to store these calories for later use. In this population in rural Guatemala it would appear that the diet is short on calories and that increasing their supply to pregnant women allows the protein in the diet or in maternal reserves to be utilized for fetal growth. This may not be true in populations where protein is the limiting dietary constituent, as in parts of Africa and Asia.

In summary, it seems clear that fetal growth is to some degree responsive to maternal nutritional status. Although maternal reserves can be utilized for fetal growth, adequate nutrition must be supplied during pregnancy. In chronically malnourished populations this is particularly true since the depleted mother has little, if any, nutritional reserve for the fetus to draw upon. We do not as yet know how much of the low birth weight in our own poor can be ascribed to inadequate maternal nutrition.

Studies by Butler in Great Britain revealed conditions similar to those described in developing countries where high and low socioeconomic groups were compared.[56] Birth weights in the lower socioeconomic groups correlated with maternal pre-pregnancy nutritional status as reflected in maternal height, whereas in both low and high socioeconomic groups there was a correlation between maternal weight gain during pregnancy and birth weight of the infant.

Basing their programs on these and other findings, a number of clinics have instituted nutritional therapy during pregnancy among the poor in the United States and Canada. Two outstanding examples are clinics in Montreal under the direction of Margaret Higgens and in San Rafael, California, under the direction of Thomas Brewer. Both have reported a marked decrease in infant mortality and morbidity as well as a significant rise in the birth weight of the infants.[54] Nevertheless, many women in the United States, some under the care of physicians, still keep their weight down during pregnancy by limiting food intake or eating foods containing less calories or protein.

In addition to the reduced survival rate of underweight infants, there is mounting evidence that those who do survive may be permanently handicapped. Data on animals and humans indicate that the consequences of malnutrition in early infancy are more severe in babies born at low weight than in those of normal weight.[58] There is also evidence that infants malnourished *in utero,* even if adequately nourished thereafter, still show certain stigmata of their intrauterine experience when they reach adulthood. In animals, for example, a derangement of nitrogen metabolism in adult life has been shown to follow fetal malnutrition. Studies in Formosa suggest that children in poor families who were undernourished in early life excrete more nitrogen than children from more affluent backgrounds.[54]

Finally, there is evidence suggesting that behavioral abnormalities may be more common in older children and adults who were malnourished *in utero* than in those whose mothers were adequately nourished. This will be discussed in detail in Chapter 5.

At this point it should be clear that malnutrition is most dangerous during the growing period. Even in its milder forms malnutrition during this period may permanently stunt growth. The possibility that it has a stunting effect on the growth of the brain which retards intellectual and behavioral development has staggering implications in view of the large number of people who have been malnourished early in life. What then are the data which demonstrate permanent effects of malnutrition on the cellular and biochemical growth and maturation of the brain? Can we document behavioral changes induced by early malnutrition? What are the implications of these changes for intellectual development? When during the growth cycle is the organism most vulnerable to nutritional deprivation? Will fetal malnutrition effect the developing brain? Is the pregnant woman vulnerable to the effects of malnutrition? All of these questions remain before us. Although all the answers are still not known we have learned a great deal. The succeeding chapters will document what we know. They paint a grim picture of a disease which is perhaps the most prevalent affliction in the world today.

REFERENCES

1. Ramalingaswami, V., Deo, M. G., Guleria, J. S., et al. Studies of the Bihar famine of 1966-67, in Symposia of the Swedish Nutrition Foundation IX, Famine, Uppsala, Almqvist & Wiksells, 1971, p. 94.
2. Smith, D. A., and Woodruff, M. F. A. Deficiency diseases in Japanese prison camps, M.R.C. Special Report Series No. 274, London, H. M. Stationery Office, 1951.
3. Edwards, R. D., and Williams, T. D. The Great Famine, Dublin, Browne and Nolan, 1956.
4. Petrides, E. P. Hunger edema in children, J. Pediatrics 32:333, 1948.
5. Lowenstein, F. W. An epidemic of kwashiorkor in South Kasai, Congo, Bull. World Health Organization 27:751, 1962.
6. Edwards, R. D., and Williams, T. D. The Great Famine, Dublin, Brown and Nolan, 1956.
7. Brown, R. E. Decreased brain weight in malnutrition and its implications, East African Med. J. 11:584, 1965.
8. Winick, M., and Rosso, P. Effects of severe early malnutrition on cellular growth of human brain, Pediat. Res. 3:181, 1969.
9. Gopolan, C. Reported at IX Int'l. Cong. Nutrition, Mexico City, 1971.
10. Chase, P., in Proc. Int'l. Cong. Pediatrics XIII, Vienna, 1971, Verlag der Wiener Medizinischen Akademie, 1971.
11. Whitehead, R. G. The causes, effects and reversibility of protein-calorie malnutrition, in Symposia of the Swedish Nutrition Foundation IX, Famine, Uppsala, Almqvist & Wiksells, 1971, p. 41.
12. Bradfield, R. B. Changes in hair associated with protein-calorie malnutrition, in Calorie Deficiencies and Protein Deficiencies, McCance, R. A., and Widdowson, E. M., eds., London, Churchill, 1968, p. 213.
13. Alleyne, G. A. O., Flores, H., Picou, D. I. M., and Waterlow, J. C. Metabolic changes in children with protein-calorie malnutrition, in Current Concepts in Nutrition, Vol. 1, Nutrition and Development, Winick, M., ed., New York, John Wiley & Sons, 1972, p. 201.

14. Ifekwunigwe, A. E. Recent field experiences in Eastern Nigeria (Biafra), in Symposia of the Swedish Nutrition Foundation IX, Famine, Uppsala, Almqvist & Wiksells, 1971, p. 144.
15. Morely, D. Measles in Nigeria, Amer. J. Dis. Child. 103:230, 1962.
16. Hendrickse, R. G. Ciba Found. Study Group, No. 31, 1967.
17. Keys, A., Brožek, J., Henschel, A., Mickelsen, O., and Taylor, A. L. The Biology of Human Starvation, Minneapolis, Univ. of Minnesota Press, 1950.
18. Whitman, W., Moodie, A. D., Hansen, J. D. L., and Brock, F. J. Ciba Found. Study Group, No. 31, 1967.
19. Foege, W. H. Famines, infections and epidemics, in Symposia of the Swedish Nutrition Foundation IX, Famine, Uppsala, Almqvist & Wiksells, 1971, p. 64.
20. Zinsser, H. Rats, Lice and History, Boston, Little, Brown and Co., 1935.
21. Prinzing, F. Epidemics Resulting from Wars, Westergaard, H., ed., Oxford, Clarendon Press, 1916.
22. Garn, S. M. Biological correlates of malnutrition in man in Nutrition, Growth and Development of North American Indian Children, Moore, W. M., Silverberg, M. M., and Read, M. S., eds., DHEW Publ. No. (NIH) 72-26, 1972, p. 129.
23. Garn, S. M. Human Races, 3rd ed., Springfield, Ill., C. C. Thomas, 1971.
24. Reisinger, K., Rogers, K. D., and Johnson, O. Nutrition survey of Lower Greasewood, Arizona Navajos, in Nutrition, Growth and Development of North American Indian Children, Moore, W. M., Silverberg, M. M., and Read, M. S., eds., DHEW Publ. No. (NIH) 72-26, 1972, p. 65.
25. Jelliffe, D. B. Infant nutrition in the subtropics and tropics, WHO Monograph Series, No. 29, Geneva, 1955.
26. Owen, G. M., Nelsen, C. E., Kram, K. M., and Garry, P. J. Nutrition survey of White Mountain Apache preschool children, in Nutrition, Growth and Development of North American Indian Children, Moore, W. M., Silverberg, M. M., and Read, M. S., eds., DHEW Publ. No. (NIH) 72-26, 1972, p. 91.
27. Winick, M., and Rosso, P. Head circumference and cellular growth of the brain in normal and marasmic children, J. Pediat. 74:774, 1969.
28. Stoch, M. B., and Smythe, P M. Does undernutrition during infancy inhibit brain growth and subsequent intellectual development, Arch. Dis. Child. 38:546, 1963.
29. Winick, M. Nutrition and mental development, Med. Cl. No. Amer. 54:1413, 1970.
30. Cravioto, J., DeLicardie, E. R., and Birch, H. G. Nutrition, growth and neurointegrative development, Pediatrics 38:319, 1966.
31. Cravioto, J., Birch, H. G., DeLicardie, E. A., and Rosales, L., The ecology of infant weight gain in a preindustrial society, Acta. Paediat. Scand. 56:71, 1967.
32. Cravioto, J., et al. The ecology of growth and development in a Mexican

preindustrial community, Soc. Res. Child Development Monograph 34, No. 5, 1969.

33. Cravioto, J. Infant malnutrition and later learning, in Progress in Human Nutrition, Margen, S., ed., Westport, Conn., The Avi Publ. Co., 1971, p. 80.

34. Manterola, A. Reported at the Latin American Society of Pediatric Research, Valdivia, Chile, 1969.

35. Sadre, M., and Donoso, G. The changing pattern of malnutrition in Iran in Progress in Human Nutrition, Vol. 1, Margen, S., ed., Westport, Conn., The Avi Publ. Co., 1971, p. 29.

36. Nutrition and Food in an African Economy, Vol. 1, Amann, V. F., Belshaw, D. G. R., and Stanfield, J. P., eds., Kampala, Uganda, Makerere Univ., April 1972.

37. Moore, W. M., Silverberg, M. M., and Read, M. S., in Nutrition, Growth and Development of North American Indian Children, eds. Ibid., DHEW Publ. No. (NIH) 72-26, 1972, p. 3.

38. Ten-State Nutrition Survey, 1968-70. DHEW Publ. No. (HSM) 72-8130-31-32-33, 1972.

39. Smith, C. A. Effects of maternal malnutrition upon the newborn infant in Holland (1944-45), Pediat. 30:229, 1947.

40. Antonov, A. N. Children born during the siege of Leningrad, J. Pediat. 30:250, 1947.

41. Newman, J. Infant Mortality: A Social Disease, London, Methuen, 1906.

42. Williams, C. D. Nutritional conditions among women and children in internment in the civilian camp at Singapore, Proc. Nutr. Soc. 5:127, 1947.

43. Kerpel-Fronius, E. Infant mortality in Budapest in the year 1945, J. Pediat. 30:244, 1947.

44. Grieve, W. P. Amenorrhea during internment, Brit. Med. J. ii, 224, 1946.

45. Hytten, F. E., and Thompson, A. M. Pregnancy, childbirth and lactation, in The Physiology of Human Survival, Edholm, O. G., and Bacharach, A. L., eds., London and New York, Academic Press, 1965, p. 327.

46. Aall, C. Relief, nutrition and health in the Nigerian/Biafran war, J. Trop. Pediat. 16:70, Monograph 9, 1970.

47. Winick, M. Cellular growth of human placenta. III. Intrauterine growth failure, J. Pediat. 71:390, 1967.

48. Winick, M., Brasel, J. A., and Velasco, E. G. Effects of prenatal nutrition upon pregnancy risk, Cl. Obstet. Gynec. 16:184, 1973.

49. Gruenwald, P., Funakawa, H., Mitani, S., Nishimura, T., and Takeuchi, S. Influence of environmental factors on foetal growth in man, Lancet 1:1026, 1967.

50. Greulich, W. W. Growth of children of the same race under different environmental conditions, Science 127:515, 1958.

51. Rush, D., Stein, Z., Christakis, G., Susser, M. The prenatal project: The first 20 months of operation, in Current Concepts in Nutrition, Vol. 2,

Nutrition and Fetal Development, Winick, M., ed., New York, John Wiley & Sons, 1974, p. 95.

52. Habicht, J-P., Yarbrough, C., Lechtig, A., and Klein, R. E. Relation of maternal supplementary feeding during pregnancy to birth weight, in Current Concepts in Nutrition, Vol. 2, Nutrition and Fetal Development, Winick, M., ed., New York, John Wiley & Sons, 1974, p. 95.

53. Alexander, S. A., and Downs, J. T. Influence of weight gain in pregnancy, Amer. J. Obstet. Gynec. 66:1161, 1953.

54. Proc. Workshop on Nutritional Suplementation and the Outcome of Pregnancy, 1971, Sagamore Beach, Mass., Washington, D.C., Nat'l Acad. Sci., 1973.

55. Thomason, A. M., and Billewicz, W. Z. Clinical significance of weight trends during pregnancy, Brit. Med. J. 1:243, 1957.

56. Butler, N. Late postnatal consequences of fetal malnutrition, in Current Concepts in Nutrition, Vol. 2, Nutrition and Fetal Development, Winick, M., ed., New York, John Wiley & Sons, 1974, p. 173.

57. Winick, M. Fetal malnutrition, Cl. Obstet. Gynec. 13:526, 1970.

Chapter 2 **NORMAL CELLULAR GROWTH OF THE BRAIN**

PRINCIPLES OF CELLULAR GROWTH

In order to understand better the mechanisms by which undernutrition exerts its effects, we must examine growth at a more fundamental level than can be done by using the methods described in Chapter 1.

Enlargement of any organ during the growing period may result from an increase in the number of cells, an increase in the size of already existing cells, or the simultaneous occurrence of both. The total number of cells can be measured by determining the total organ DNA content and then dividing by a constant which represents the DNA content per diploid nucleus in the species being studied.[1, 2] This constant has been determined for a variety of species. In the rat, all diploid cells contain 6.2 pg of DNA; in the human all diploid cells contain 6.0 pg of DNA. With the exception of a few tetraploid Purkinje cells in the cerebellum and in the cerebral cortex, all of the cells making up the mammalian brain are diploid.[3] Therefore, the DNA content of the brain accurately reflects the total number of cells. Similarly, the DNA content of the various brain regions represents the total number of cells in each area. In the liver, the existence of polyploidy makes these measurements more difficult to interpret; however, it has been shown that as ploidy increases the cytoplasmic mass of the cell increases proportionally.[4] A tetraploid liver cell nucleus therefore governs twice as much cytoplasm as a diploid liver nucleus. Thus, liver growth can be examined by the same method as long as one remembers that although a doubling of the chromosome number will double the nuclear DNA content, it may not result in two discrete nuclei. The cytoplasm will also double in size but will not divide into two separate cells.

Certain other organs such as skeletal muscle and aging pancreas contain a significant proportion of multinuclear cells.[5] In these organs an increase in DNA content represents an increase in nuclear number and not an increase in the actual number of cells. If one assumes that each nucleus governs a discrete, though not bounded, cytoplasmic mass, then again the same principles may be employed. Finally, certain organs contain diploid nuclei but no discrete cell boundaries (syncytia). Placenta in most species is such an organ. Again, the same principles can be used to determine cell numbers in these organs if we assume that each nucleus governs a discrete cytoplasmic mass.

After we have determined the number of cells using this biochemical approach, the average weight per cell, protein content per cell, RNA content per cell, and lipid content per cell can be determined simply by analyzing for the total amount of each of these components and dividing by the number of cells. The result can be expressed chemically as a weight/DNA, protein/DNA, RNA/DNA, or lipid/DNA ratio. Thus, regardless of whether actual cell number or "cell mass" is calculated, the thesis that an increase in total organ DNA content represents one aspect of growth, namely, an increase in the number of cells, would appear valid. Increases in the weight/DNA or protein/DNA ratio and, in certain cases, the lipid/DNA ratio represent another aspect of growth, namely, increase in cell size.

It should be noted that total DNA content, while accurately reflecting cell number, of course in no way differentiates one cell type from another. In addition, although the ratios mentioned above give an over-all average for each component per cell, not a single cell may actually contain this average quantity of material. Individual cells, especially when differing in type, may vary widely in their composition of protein, RNA, or lipids. This is particularly true in the central nervous system which is made up of a variety of cell types of different sizes and shapes. Although functionally these cells can be divided into neurons and glia, there is considerable variation within these categories. For example, the large cerebral neurons differ from the small cerebellar neurons, and astrocytes differ markedly from oligodendroglia in size and shape. In addition, there are supporting cells connected with the blood vessels, and cells of the vasculature itself. All of these cell types contribute to the over-all cellular makeup of the brain. The fact that methods just described do not differentiate among them has limited the scope of information such studies can provide. Within this limitation, however, the "chemical" approach to growth has allowed us to make certain generalizations which give a broad picture of growth at a cellular level.

Early growth in the organs of the rat proceeds entirely by cell division. Weight, protein, and DNA all increase proportionally. This results in constant cell size expressed either as a weight/DNA or a protein/DNA ratio.[6] The rate of DNA synthesis, and therefore of cell division, decreases at different times for different organs. Protein content, however, continues to rise, resulting in an increased protein/DNA ratio. Increase in cell size, then, occurs as a consequence not of increased rates of protein accumulation, but of decreased rates of DNA synthesis or cell division. If the weight/DNA ratio is used to assess cell size, the same relationships hold as for protein, except during the neonatal period, when weight/DNA ratios either remain constant or decrease. This suggests that a loss of water occurs during the neonatal period, an observation that has been made in man and many animals.[7]

Growth begins to slow down as maturity is approached and this slowing is due to attainment of a steady state between protein synthesis and degradation. It should be noted that DNA synthesis stops in most organs before the organ has attained its maximum weight or protein content.[6] For the rat and most of its organs, growth from 10 days after conception to maturity can be divided into three phases. In the first phase there is rapid cell division with cell size remaining constant. In the second both cell number and cell size increase as DNA and protein content rise, but, because of a decrease in the rate of DNA synthesis, protein rises out of proportion to DNA. In the third there is an increase in cell size as DNA synthesis stops and protein continues to accumulate. Growth finally ceases when protein synthesis and degradation come into equilibrium. These phases do not change abruptly but merge gradually, one into the other (Fig. 2-1).

The organs of the lymphoid system show an entirely different pattern of growth. In both spleen and thymus, weight/DNA and protein/DNA ratios remain constant. Growth in these organs occurs by cell division without increase in cell size. It is interesting that of all the organs studied these two are the only ones of the so-called renewing type with a rapid cell turnover.

Total organ RNA content increases progressively during growth. Except in liver, this increase is always proportional to the increase in DNA, resulting in an RNA/DNA ratio that is constant in the particular organ

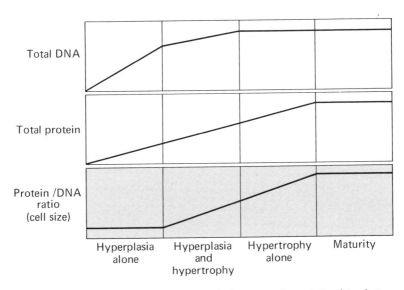

Fig. 2.1. Periods of cellular growth. Plotted above are the relationships between DNA and protein during the three phases of organ growth. It will be observed that DNA content crests and levels off well before organ size, as determined by protein accretion, and weight gain, reaches its maximum.

and does not vary with time. Certain tissues such as liver, heart, and skeletal muscle show a high RNA/DNA ratio, whereas tissues such as spleen and thymus show low ratios. These data tend to reinforce the concept that tissues most actively engaged in protein synthesis are rich in RNA. A high RNA/DNA ratio, however, occurs early in development, before the high protein/DNA ratios are reached in the same tissues. Skeletal muscle, heart, and salivary gland are good examples of this phenomenon. RNA/DNA ratios are high but do not change significantly from 4 to 44 days. Protein/DNA ratios, however, increase markedly during that period (Fig. 2-2). It appears that during early growth RNA reaches its final amount per cell even in the face of rapid cell division and that this amount is sufficient to sustain normal rates of protein synthesis.[6] Liver appears to be one exception. Our data indicate an increase in the RNA/DNA ratio in liver during the neonatal period, a change which correlates with the increased enzymatic activity occurring in liver at that time.

We can now view the over-all growth of an organ as a continuous accretion of protoplasm made up of water, proteins, RNA, and in some

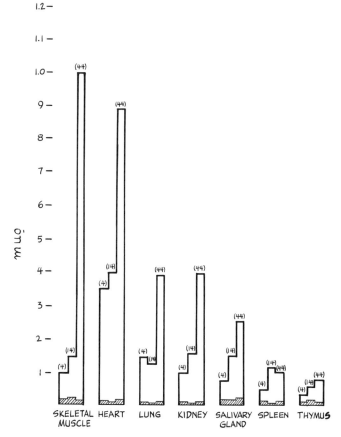

Fig. 2.2. Comparison of RNA and protein per nucleus during normal growth in the rat. ( ) = days after birth; □ = protein per nucleus; ▨ = RNA per nucleus.

cases lipids. The ultimate arrangement of this protoplasm into individual cells depends on the rate of DNA synthesis. The mechanisms controlling the period during which DNA may be synthesized by an organ and those governing the rate of synthesis during that period are largely unknown, but in recent years some insight into these mechanisms has been achieved. The time during organ growth when cells are actively proliferating is under genetic control. This time will vary tremendously in different species. For example in the rat brain, cell division is over by the twenty-first postnatal day.[6] In the guinea pig there is very little cell division in brain after birth. By contrast, in the human brain, cell division continues through the first year of life[8] (Fig 2-3).

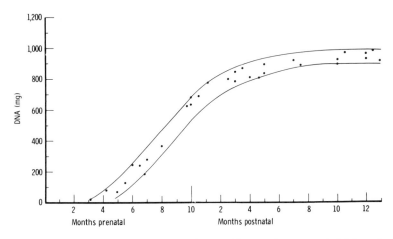

Fig. 2.3. Amount of DNA in the brain of normal human fetuses and children. Each dot represents one brain.

BRAIN

In this section we will discuss a number of the major biochemical events in brain tissue and how they change during development. The processes to be considered are those which are influenced by the nutritional status of the organism: the number, size, and type of cells; myelination and lipid metabolism; the metabolism of carbohydrates; the transport and utilization of amino acids; and the synthesis and degradation of proteins. Although we will discuss each of these major processes separately, it must be remembered that many are occurring simultaneously and developmental changes in one area are often prerequisites of changes in other areas.

The number, type, and size of cells

Detailed examination of normal cellular growth in the rat brain reveals that different regions undergo different patterns of growth. For example, in cerebrum DNA synthesis continues until about 21 days postnatally.[9] After 21 days the cells continue to accumulate protein and lipid. Thus, total cerebral lipid content is achieved at about 65 days and total protein content at about 99 days of age. In cerebellum, the synthesis of DNA stops at about 17 days postnatally.[10] After this, net protein synthesis actually declines for a short period of time and the size of the individual cerebellar cells decreases. This reduction in the size of the individual cells of the cerebellum with age probably reflects the maturation of larger, more primitive cerebellar cells into smaller, more mature cells. In brain stem, the total number of cells increases until about 14 days of age. After this there is an enormous increase in the protein/DNA ratio. This increase probably reflects an increase not only in the size of the brain stem cells themselves but also in growth, myelination, and extension of neuronal processes from other brain regions into the brain stem. Cellular growth in the hippocampus is unique to the central nervous system. Although one can demonstrate a very discrete rise in DNA content between the fourteenth and the seventeenth day of life,[10] this does not correspond to an increase in the rate of cell division within the hippocampus but rather to a migration of neurons from under the lateral ventricle into the hippocampus which occurs precisely on the fifteenth day of life in the rat.[11, 12] Figure 2-4 illustrates the changes in DNA content in various regions of the rat brain with age.

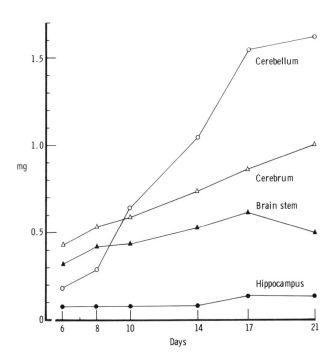

Fig. 2.4. Total DNA content in various regions of rat brain

The cellular makeup of any region of the brain depends on the rate of cell division within the region, on the time that cell division normally stops in that region, on the types of cells which are undergoing division at that particular time, and on whether or not cells are migrating to or from the region. In extensive autoradiographic studies it has been demonstrated that neuronal cell division in rat cerebrum ceases before birth. In cerebellum, however, both neuronal and glial precursors of all cell types continue to divide in the postnatal period. There is also active proliferation of cells under the third and fourth ventricles.[13] The cells under the fourth ventricle migrate to the hippocampus on precisely the fifteenth postnatal day.[12] Less is known about brain development in other species. In the pig, the most rapid rate of cell division is around birth; in the guinea pig and subhuman primate it is before birth.[14] Regional patterns have not yet been described in these animals although extensive histochemical studies during development have been carried out in the squirrel monkey.[15]

Patterns of cellular growth are not nearly so well defined in the human brain as in the rat brain.[8, 16, 17] Studies in our laboratory indicated that DNA synthesis is linear prenatally, begins to slow down shortly after birth, and reaches a maximum at about 8 to 12 months of age[8] (Fig. 2-3). More recent studies have modified these results somewhat and extend the time beyond the first year of life.[16, 18] Moreover, Dobbing and Sands have shown that there are two peaks of DNA synthesis which occur normally during the development of the human brain. The first peak is reached at about 26 weeks of gestation and the second peak around birth (Fig. 2-5).[18] These authors have interpreted their results as corresponding to the peak rate of neuronal division and the peak rate of glial division, respectively. It must be understood, however, that although this interpretation would fit the known data from other studies of human brain development, no direct evidence pinpointing the cell types involved has been found.

There is still very little evidence about the cellular growth of the various regions of the human brain. Available data indicate that the rate of cell division postnatally is about the same in cerebrum and cerebellum and that cell division stops at about the same time in both areas, that is, between 12 and 15 months of age[19] (Fig. 2-6). However, the number of cases studied is too small to determine the exact time at which cell division stops in these areas. In brain stem, DNA synthesis continues at a slow but steady rate until at least 1 year of age.[19] Here again, the cell

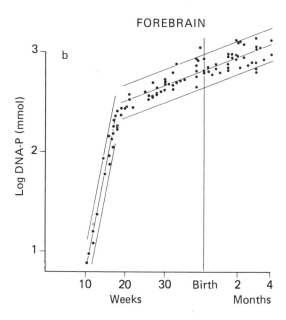

Fig. 2.5.   DNA content of human fetal brain

types involved and the migratory patterns of the cells in the developing human brain are not as clearly understood as in the rat brain. For obvious reasons, autoradiography cannot be done. What we do know about the human brain is the result of careful histological and histochemical examination of brains of fetuses of various ages. In a series of elegant studies, Duckett and Pearse have shown that during fetal life the brain not only increases linearly in weight but undergoes a series of complicated biochemical changes.[20, 21, 22, 23] Glycolysis is present during the second month of fetal life; oxidative mechanisms appear during the third month; and activity and localization of a number of enzymes reach a mature pattern during the seventh month of fetal life. The presence of acetylcholinesterase has been thought to indicate tissue excitability.[24] The activity of this enzyme is localized in neurons of the anterior horn of the spinal cord as early as the tenth week of embryonic life. This correlates well with the time when movement of the lower limb can be elicited by proper stimulation.[25] These data become more interesting when coupled with the developmental pattern of acetylcholinesterase in

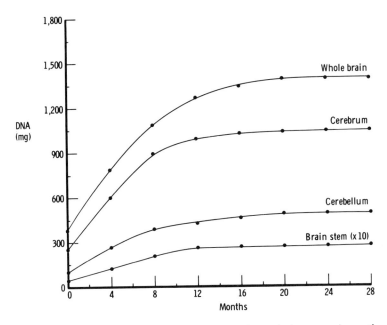

Fig. 2.6. DNA content in various regions of human brain during normal growth

the rat brain, since it has been shown in the rat that the activity of acetyl-cholinesterase can be altered by malnutrition occurring early in life.[26]

Two specific cell types, the Cajal-Retzius cells and the monamine oxidase cells, are present only in fetal life, disappearing before birth.[21, 22] Their function is unknown, and the mechanisms responsible for both their appearance and disappearance have not been adequately studied.

Myelination and lipid metabolism

Not only is the brain composed of a multiplicity of cell types, but many of the cells of the brain contain relatively large amounts of lipid. The major components of brain lipids are both simple lipids such as cholesterol and fatty acids and compound lipids such as phospholipids, glycolipids, and other esters. Although most of the lipid is contained within cell membranes, e.g., myelin sheaths, some is contained in other subcellular fractions, such as endoplasmic reticulum and mitochondria. Since the bulk of the total brain lipid is present as a component of myelin, lipid changes during development constitute changes in myelination.

Cholesterol is the only sterol present in appreciable amounts in the adult nervous system. In the young animal, however, demosterol and zymosterol have been reported.[27, 28] These appear to be precursors of cholesterol. Although most cholesterol in the nervous system is in the free form, fatty esters of cholesterol are also present, especially in the young animal.[29] There are some data to suggest that another cholesterol ester, cholesterol sulfate, is also present in the normal brain.[30] Only trace amounts of free fatty acids are present in brain; the bulk of the fatty acids exist as esters of compound lipids.[31] Phospholipids, which account for 20 to 25% of the dry weight of mammalian brain, are compounds in which phosphatidic acid is combined with a base (either choline or ethanolamine) and a hydroxyamino acid (serine or inositol). Phospholipids include lecithins (phosphatidyl choline), cephalins (phosphatidyl ethanolamine), lipositols (phosphatidyl inositol), phosphatidyl serine, plasmalogens (acetal phosphatide), and sphingomyelins (phosphatidyl sphingosides).

Sphingomyelin is the major phosphosphingolipid in animal tissues. Although it contains phosphorylcholine, it differs from lecithin in that the fatty acid is bound by an amide linkage to sphingosine. The di-phosphoinositides and triphosphoinositides, although present in only small amounts, are important in assessing myelination since they are highly concentrated in the myelin sheath.

Glycolipids exist in the brain primarily in two forms, cerebrosides or cerebroside sulfates (sulfatides), and gangliosides. Cerebrosides contain galactose, a high-molecular-weight fatty acid, and sphingol or sphingosine (the same complex aminoalcohol that is present in sphingomyelin). In the adult brain 90% of the total cerebroside is located within the myelin sheath. Gangliosides are present in lower concentration than cerebrosides. They consist of *N*-acetyl neuraminic acid, sphingosine, and three molecules of either glucose or galactose. Gangliosides are found mainly in those areas containing neurons and are concentrated at nerve endings.[32] For this reason the ganglioside concentration has been taken by some to reflect the number of neurons present in any given area. In addition, since the highest concentration of gangliosides is at the dendridic tips, the amount of this lipid has been used by some investigators as a measure of dendritic arborization.[33]

Total lipid content and concentration increase in the whole brain during development. The major increase in concentration occurs in white matter rather than in gray matter. Undoubtedly this is because progressive myelination is occurring primarily in the white matter. The rate of total lipid deposition can be used to measure the rate of myelin synthesis because of the very low turnover in the components of myelin in all mammalian species thus far studied.[34] In this respect myelin resembles DNA as described previously. Investigators have generaliy found a marked increase in the total lipid content and concentration during the early development of the brain in most mammalian species including man.[35] The developmental changes in the major lipid components of the rat brain are summarized in Table 2-1. The rate of cholesterol deposition is maximal between the fifteenth and twentieth days of postnatal growth. This is about one week after the DNA synthesis peaks.[14]

In the human brain there is little change in total lipid composition in either gray or white matter during the first 7 months of gestation. Thereafter, lipid deposition proceeds rapidly in gray matter until adult composition is reached at about three months of age. In white matter, where most of the actual myelination occurs, there is a much less rapid deposition of lipids. By 2 years of age, however, 90% of the total lipid has been deposited and by 10 years of age adult values have been attained.[36, 37, 38]

Cholesterol concentration begins to increase in cerebral gray and white matter and in cerebellum early in fetal life.[39] In whole brains of fetuses under 2 months of age cholesterol concentration is 2.4%. This concen-

Table 2-1
CHANGES IN LIPID COMPOSITION
OF THE DEVELOPING RAT BRAIN

	Age (days)	Wet Weight (g)	Cholesterol (mmoles)	Phospholipid (mmoles)	Cerebrosides (mmoles)	Molar Ratio Cholesterol: Phospholipid: Cerebrosides
Whole brain	10	1.00	16.00	33.60	0.18	100:210:1
	16	1.25	26.90	53.00	1.25	100:197:4.5
	Adult	1.99	96.00	119.00	22.20	100:125:23
Myelin	10	1.00	1.47	2.07	0.077	100:140:5
	16	—	3.20	4.47	0.320	100:140:10
	Adult	—	34.0	32.0	11.8	100:95:35

Reprinted from *Applied Neurochemistry*. A. N. Davison and J. Dobbing, eds. Blackwell Scientific Publications, Oxford and Edinburgh, 1968, p. 273.

tration rises to 5.4% at birth, 6.65% by 9 months of age, and 10.7% in the adult brain.[36] Data on cerebrosides are not clear but suggest an increased concentration in white matter during normal development.[38] In all of the phospholipid fractions there is an increase in concentration during development. Phosphatides show very little increase after seven months' gestation.[36, 38] In contrast, cephalin concentration in white and gray matter increases from 7% at 4 months' gestation to 12% in gray matter and 17% in white matter, which are the adult levels, by 3 months of postnatal age.

Myelination is always preceded by the multiplication of oligodendroglial cells.[40] After this has occurred, the glial cells surround the nerve axon in a spiral fashion. When this "wrapping" process is completed, a progressive deposition of lipids begins within the myelin sheath.[41] Lipids represent about 75% of the dry weight of human myelin. The largest lipid component is cholesterol, but significant amounts of ethanolamine phosphatide, galactolipids, cerebrosides, and cerebroside sulfates are present. The characteristic composition of myelin lipids in the human shows a molar ratio of cholesterol : phospholipid : cerebroside of 2 : 2 : 1.

Studies of myelin composition during development have demonstrated that considerable changes take place in the lipid composition as myelin deposition progresses. The concentration of lecithin decreases when compared to that of other phospholipids. By contrast, cholesterol, phosphatidyl inositol, and ethanolamine phosphatide increase in comparison to other lipid components.

Myelin itself cannot be considered a discrete metabolic entity. Experiments employing C^{14} labeling have shown that acetic inositol phosphatide, lecithin, and serine phosphatide have much more rapid turnover rates than most of the other components, which show very slow rates of turnover.[14] Despite its relative nonspecificity, however, cholesterol content has been used in assessing myelination because of its very slow turnover rate and also because it is so easy to measure.

Serial analysis of lipids in human brains indicates that the lipid/DNA ratio (the amount of lipid per cell) rises from shortly after birth until at least 2 years of age (Fig. 2-7). This increase is reflected in a rise in both the cholesterol/DNA ratio and the phospholipid/DNA ratio. Thus, postnatal lipid synthesis is proceeding at a more rapid rate than DNA synthesis, undoubtedly as a result of the rapid myelination that is occurring during this period of life as well as the decrease in the rate of cell division which begins then.[42]

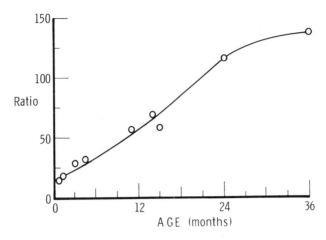

Fig. 2.7. Lipid-DNA ratio in normal children at different ages

The metabolism of carbohydrates

Recent studies in developing rat brain have shown that during the period of most rapid lipid synthesis, glucose is metabolized in much greater proportion through the hexose monophosphate shunt than it is later. More than 50% of glucose metabolism is carried through this pathway until about 30 days of age; thereafter less than 20% of the metabolism of glucose goes through the shunt[13] (Fig. 2-8). Although the reasons for this relative shift in pathways are unknown, the hexose monophosphate shunt favors both nucleic acid and lipid synthesis. For the former it supplies ribose molecules, and for the latter it generates TPNH. Human brain has not been studied in this respect. It would be interesting to know whether more glucose is metabolized via the hexose monophosphate shunt pathway in infant brain than in adult brain, especially during those periods in human brain growth when proliferation of cells and deposition of myelin are occurring.

Glucose is of course the predominant substrate utilized by the brain under normal conditions. It is almost totally metabolized to CO_2 and lactate. The evidence for this comes from a number of sources: first, the respiratory quotient of brain is approximately 1.0; second, glucose is the only metabolite extracted from the blood by brain tissue in sufficient amounts to account for this respiratory rate; third, the reduction in the supply of glucose to the brain results in a decrease in the respiratory rate as well as an impairment in cerebral function.[43]

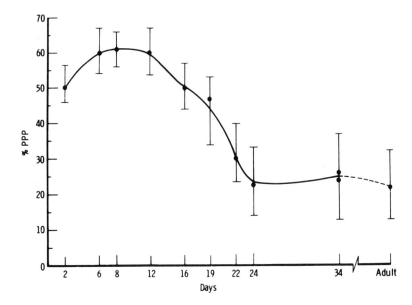

Fig. 2.8. Percent of total gluscose metabolized through the hexosemonophosphate shunt in normal rat brain

During development, as we shall see, certain biochemical processes are exceedingly sensitive to the nutritional state of the animal. The effects of undernutrition on brain respiratory rate have been studied recently as one indicator of the damage produced by early undernutrition.[44]

In most species, the rate of glucose utilization in the adult brain is 0.3–1.0 mmol/kg/min, and more than 90% of the glucose consumed is metabolized via the glycolytic pathway. Under normal conditions, only a small fraction of the pyruvate formed is converted to lactate; the rest is oxidized, within the mitochondria, via the citric acid cycle to CO_2 and H_2O. Both glycolysis and pyruvate oxidation are very efficient, conserving energy in the form of ATP. The quantity of ATP present in the brain at any point in time reflects the amount of stored energy at that time. Changes in ATP content of the brain during normal development have not been carefully studied; however, attempts have been made recently to study the effects of undernutrition early in life on ATP content of the developing brain. To date no changes have been found, suggesting that energy stored in this manner is conserved extremely well.[45]

The unique position of glucose in brain metabolism is at least in part related to the fact that most other compounds cross the "blood-brain barrier" only with difficulty. Observations on this barrier, however, have been made mostly in adult animals; its development during early life has not been carefully studied in relation to many substances. It is not known whether the barrier develops at the same time for all substances or whether permeability to individual substances changes at different rates. This is an area of research that may yield important information regarding the effects of early malnutrition on the central nervous system.

Certain other metabolic pathways are present in the brain, including a modification of the Krebs cycle known as the γ-amino-butyrate (GABA) shunt.[46] The succinyl-CoA step in the Krebs cycle may be bypassed by this pathway. Although the presence of the GABA shunt can be clearly demonstrated *in vivo,* its quantitative importance is unknown.[47] In the adult guinea pig cortex, estimates indicate that it accounts for about 10% of the total turnover of glucose.[48] The pathway provides an alternative direction from glutamate to aspartate, through oxaloacetate, or from γ-oxoglutarate to succinate.[49] Its time of appearance and functional importance during development have not yet been studied. Nor have the effects of environmental alterations or altered nutritional status on the amount of glucose shunted in and out of this pathway yet been examined.

When the availability of oxygen to the adult brain is reduced, the only significant sources of energy are ATP, phosphocreatine, and high energy phosphate bonds formed by the conversion of glucose and glycogen to lactate. When such reduction occurs, the rate of glucose and phosphocreatine consumption exceeds that of glycogen and ATP, but all available sources are depleted within two to three minutes. Again, little is known about sources of energy in the developing brain. The newborn mammalian brain, including the human brain, will withstand hypoxia for a longer period of time than the adult brain. Just why this is so, however, remains unknown. By contrast, recent experiments indicate that even relatively short periods of hypoxia will reduce the rate of cell division, as measured by total DNA content and by thymidine incorporation studies in neonatal rat brain.[50] The newborn then may tolerate anoxic periods but cell division will be impaired. This is extremely important in that form of "fetal malnutrition" which involves vascular insufficiency to the developing fetus. This type of malnutrition results not only in a decrease in nutrients of the conventional type but also in a decrease in oxygen.

During development, a change in the relative importance of glycolysis versus respiration occurs in brain tissue. For example, the brain of 4- to 6-day-old chick embryos already contains energy-rich phosphate and exhibits both glycolysis and respiration. In the mammal, glycolysis predominates during the early stages of brain development. After birth, respiration becomes more and more important until it assumes the dominant role in glucose metabolism. This change does not take place uniformly throughout the brain but proceeds in a caudocephalic direction, from the spinal cord to the cerebral cortex.[43] It would certainly seem logical to assume that the relative insensitivity which the infant brain exhibits to anoxia in terms of energy depletion is in some way linked to its normal reliance more on glycolysis than on respiration.

Since glycogen has a relatively rapid turnover rate, it must be regarded as a dynamic component of the nervous system. It is present in both neuronal and glial elements,[43] but its role during development in adult life is unknown.

The transport and utilization of amino acids

Amino acids are supplied to the nervous system by the blood, which acts as a reservoir from which these acids are removed by the activity of the tissues it supplies. The amino acids move from this reservoir into the interior of the cell through the capillary wall and the cell membrane. The membranes of nerve cells contain a number of transport systems for specific groups of amino acids, and it is these transport systems which regulate the flow of amino acids into and out of the cells. Most of the studies designed to explore the mechanisms involved in amino acid transport have been carried out on tissue slices, which are able to concentrate amino acids against a concentration gradient. When experiments are conducted with intact animals, amino acids are concentrated by adult brain much less well. These differences between the *in vitro* and *in vivo* experiments have been partially responsible for the development of the concept of a blood brain barrier—a concept which is being questioned at present. The *in vitro* experiments, however, clearly demonstrate that brain tissue has the capacity to concentrate various amino acids against a concentration gradient and that this transport is reduced by oxygen restriction and by metabolic inhibitors.[51, 52, 53]

Upon entry into the cell, amino acids undergo a number of alterations through such processes as transamination, deamination, decarboxylation, or hydroxylation, thus forming new compounds. Studies of these enzymatic conversions in brain tissue have not been numerous, but there is considerable information about the amino acids involved in certain pharmacological or neurotransmitter functions such as dihydroxyphenylalanine (DOPA), 5-hydroxytryptamine, and histidine. The enzymes involved in these conversions exhibit specific developmental patterns and recent studies have shown that their activity may be altered by early malnutrition.[54]

Most of the amino acids within brain tissue are synthesized from glucose. After adding uniformly labeled C^{14} glucose to a medium containing rat cerebral cortex, a significant amount of radioactivity can be recovered from the amino acid pool within 60 minutes. The major portion of this radioactivity is present in glutamate and two of its products, glutamine and GABA. In addition, aspartate and alanine are also labeled.[55] Thus, those amino acids linked to glucose through the Krebs cycle can be synthesized from glucose. Figure 2-9 outlines the central pathways of glucose metabolism and the interrelation between glutamate, glutamine, alanine, and the Krebs cycle. Glutamate occupies a central position. It is present in high concentration. It can take part in numerous reactions and can be oxidized at a relatively high rate. In addition, glutamate can be formed from GABA by transamination. Moreover, glutamate may be combined with ammonium ions by glutamine synthetase to form glutamine. In the brain this reaction appears to be reversible and thereby provides a mechanism for the removal of ammonia.[56] Glutamate may also be decarboxylated to form GABA and subsequently metabolized, as pre-

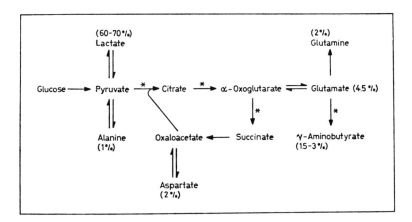

Fig. 2.9. Central pathways of glucose metabolism

viously mentioned. Finally, glutamate is in reversible equilibrium with γ-oxoglutarate and therefore provides an egress from and an entry into the Krebs cycle. Glucose, pyruvate and carbon dioxide thus can contribute to the formation of dicarboxylic acid and other amino acids in the brain by way of this cycle. This has been repeatedly demonstrated by administering isotopically labeled glucose *in vivo* and recovering significant radioactivity in the free amino acid pool as aspartate, glutamate, glutamine, glutathione, *N*-acetyl-aspartate, and GABA. It has also been shown that lowering brain glucose concentration either *in vivo* or *in vitro* results in a reduction in the concentration of glutamate, glutamine, GABA, alanine, and glycine.[57, 58, 59]

Another extremely important substance in brain metabolism is γ-amino butyric acid (GABA). Figure 2-10 depicts the pathways of

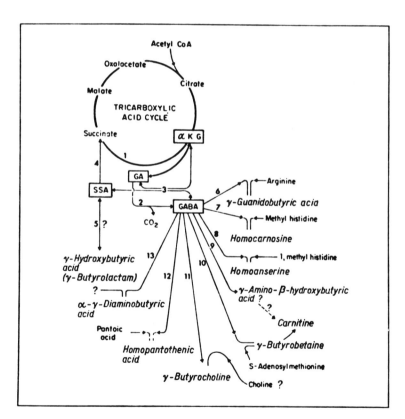

Fig. 2.10. Pathways of GABA, gamma amino buteric acid, metabolism in mammalian brain

GABA metabolism in mammalian brain. Pathways 2, 3, and 4 represent the GABA shunt around the Krebs cycle (pathway 1). Pathways 6 to 13 represent alternate routes of GABA utilization. GABA-transaminase, which gives rise to succinate, is the major pathway by which GABA is metabolized. It is not the only pathway, however, and through the others such products as guanido-butyric acid (GABA-arginine), homocarnosine (GABA histidine) homoanerserine (GABA-1-methyl-histidine), γ-butyro-betaine, carnitine, and γ-amino-butyl-choline are formed. The formation of these products, which are almost unique in the nervous system, may be one of GABA's key roles, although at present the function of most of them is unknown.

Glycine, another amino acid which has recently achieved prominence, may be a neurotransmitter in the spinal cord.[60] It is synthesized from glucose via D-3-phosphoglyceric acid and serine. Labeled glucose is rapidly converted *in vivo* into serine, alanine, and glycine. In nervous tissue glucose is converted to serine mainly through the "phosphorylated" route in which phosphoglyceric acid dehydrogenase is a catalyst.[61] Serine can then be converted to glycine in the presence of transhydroxymethylase, a folic acid dependent enzyme. The exact function of glycine and the pathways of its metabolism are still being investigated, as are the factors involved in regulating its concentration.

Another group of amino acids is essential to central nervous system metabolism. These include 5-hydroxytryptophane, DOPA, and histidine, which act as precursors for the amines 5-hydroxytryptamine (serotonin), dopamine, norepinephrine, and histamine. These compounds are of major significance in neurotransmission and they exhibit specific developmental patterns which can be altered by early malnutrition.[54] It is known that norepinephrine concentration in the rat brain increases after birth, reaching a maximum at about 8 days of age.[62] Malnutrition imposed during this period of rapid norepinephrine increase will result in a curtailment of that increase and a reduction in the amount of norepinephrine within the brain.[63] There have been similar findings regarding serotonin.[63]

The level of free amino acids in nervous tissue is relatively stable even under a variety of adverse conditions. Under conditions altering the Krebs cycle, however, concentration of certain amino acids, particularly glutamic and aspartic acids, GABA, glutamine, and alanine, may be changed. Removal of a given amino acid from the diet will also lower its concentration in nervous tissue.[64] The significance of these observations during development in malnourished animals has not yet been assessed.

In general, 8 amino acids (lysine, threonine, tryptophane, methionine, phenylalanine, leucine, valine, and isoleucine) are required for both growth and nitrogen balance by all mammalian species. In addition, arginine is considered essential to all species except the adult rat, mouse, dog, and man. Not only will deficiencies of these amino acids alter metabolism, but their administration in disproportionate amounts will also lead to metabolic difficulties.[65, 66] In yet another reminder of the current boundaries of our knowledge, it must be said that amino acid requirements of the developing nervous system are not known.

The synthesis and degradation of proteins

The major role of amino acids in the brain, as in all other tissues, is to form protein. In the past it was thought that central nervous system proteins were metabolically quite stable, with little or no turnover of the constituent amino acids. More recent studies indicate that quite the contrary is true.[67, 68, 69] Brain protein molecules are in a dynamic state with respect to their constituent amino acids, which are constantly moving into and coming out of the protein molecules. The rate of turnover varies in different brain regions and with different types of protein. Turnover of proteolipids, for example, is relatively slow compared with the turnover of other proteins.

Protein turnover is of course an outcome of the synthesis and degradation of protein that is constantly occurring. Studies of the degradative enzymes, especially those in cell membranes, have been extensive. Neutral proteinase enzymes have been detected in both the central and the peripheral nervous system.[70, 71] They are localized in mitochondria and myelin and their exact role in protein metabolism is unknown. There are some indications that these enzymes might play a role in membrane transport as well as protein turnover.

Generally speaking, the mechanisms involved in protein synthesis seem to be similar in all tissues, including the brain. Protein is synthesized primarily on the cytoplasmic ribosome but also to some extent on "ribosomes" or RNA-containing structures within the nucleus, mitochondria, and, probably, nerve endings.

During development it is possible to study protein synthesis by exam-

ining variations in the concentration and activity of amino acid incorporating systems in brain cells. Studies of this type have demonstrated
that over-all protein synthesis is more active in the immature brain than
in the adult brain. At present, however, we do not know the relative con-
tributions of different cell types and subcellular structures to this pattern.
The average half-life of proteins in rat brain increases with age as a consequence of an accentuated synthesis of proteins with long turnover
rates.[68] There is a rapid decline in the rate of protein synthesis in cerebral
cortex soon after birth and a more gradual decline thereafter.[72] In addition, proteins of all subcellular fractions are more highly labeled after
injection of a radioactive precursor in young rat brain than in adult rat
brain, indicating that this decline in protein synthesis occurs in all of the
cell fractions where protein is being synthesized.[73, 74] Other *in vitro* and
in vivo experiments support the conclusion that the rate of over-all synthesis in brain declines with age. For example, cortical slices from 16-
day-old rats incorporate ^{14}C-valine into protein at one-sixth the rate of
cortical slices from 7-day-old rats.[75] One of the explanations put forth
for this reduction in protein-synthesizing activity which occurs with maturation of the brain is a change in the ribosomal patterns and/or in ac-
tivating enzymes. Recently it has been shown that preparations from the
cerebral cortex of newborn or 2-day-old rats contain significantly higher
proportions of polysomes than corresponding preparations from the cerebral cortex of either 22-day-old or adult animals.[69] This change with age
in the direction of smaller aggregates of ribosomes is accompanied by
reductions in the amino acid incorporating ability of the tissues. Our
present understanding of protein synthesis suggests that it is carried out
more effectively on larger polysomes and thus this shift to smaller aggregates would be quite consistent with the other evidence suggesting
reduced protein synthesis with maturation. It has been clearly demonstrated, both *in vitro* and *in vivo,* that malnutrition will shift the polysome pattern in rat liver in the direction of smaller aggregates.[76]

An indication of the rate of protein synthesis *in vivo* has been derived
from turnover studies. The mean half-life of proteins in the rat brain is
17 days, but recent experiments have shown that turnover of individual
proteins may vary widely. Some have a mean half-life as short as 3 or 4
days.[43] There is no direct evidence about the *in vivo* rate of protein synthesis in the human brain, but estimates based on a mean half-life of 14
days would indicate an over-all synthesis of at least four grams of protein per day. This represents a rate of protein synthesis similar to that of

secreting glandular tissue. The rate in brain tissue is undoubtedly greater than in muscle and most other organs and may be related in some way to the functional activity of the neurons.

Proteins are indirectly synthesized *in vivo* from glucose. As mentioned earlier in this chapter, the glucose carbon is transferred to the glutamate pool, which is relatively large in the brain and which may give rise to other amino acids and, therefore, to proteins.

If these metabolic characteristics of the brain are of functional significance, this would be revealed by the metabolic changes occurring at the time during development when functional activity first begins. Various studies have shown that the metabolism of glucose in fetal and immature rat brain is similar to that of other organs. The rapid conversion of glucose carbon into amino acids, which is characteristic of the adult brain, is absent up to 10-12 days after birth, but develops quickly during the critical phase in the growth and development of the brain, when the cerebral cortex becomes functionally mature.[43] At that time there is an increase in the synthesis of new protein, an increase in the activity of enzymes related to synaptic transmission, and also a net increase in the conversion of glucose into carboxylic acid and other compounds.

In summary, we can see that brain growth is characterized by proliferation of various cell types. Each cell type multiplies most rapidly in a given area at a given time. In general neurons increase fastest early in development whereas glial multiplication is most rapid later. Cerebellar proliferation in rat brain is more rapid than cerebral proliferation postnatally. There are not enough data to be sure of these relative rates in the human brain. Following this period of active proliferation is the period of most active myelin deposition. This entails not only changes in the content of various lipids indicating a progressive increase in the amount of myelin but also changes in the concentrations of various lipids which indicates changes in the composition of the myelin being deposited. Certain specific lipids such as gangliosides increase during this period, suggesting an increase in the number of dendrites and hence by inference in the number of synapses.

Glucose is metabolized during early development via pathways most efficient for the developing brain. The hexosemonophosphate shunt is active, favoring lipid and nucleic acid synthesis. The capability to convert glucose to amino acids is present early in development. Amino acids are used for protein synthesis and for the synthesis of a number of specialized compounds which act as chemical transmitters of nerve impulses.

Not only are the amino acids available for protein synthesis but the apparatus necessary to synthesize proteins develops early and progresses more efficiently. For example, there is an increase in polyribosomes as the brain matures. An increased proportion of polyribosomes indicates more efficient protein synthesis.

It must be noted that there is still much to be learned about the normal biochemical development of the brain. Perhaps our need for information is greatest in regard to the relationship between these biochemical events and the function of nervous tissue, even at its most primitive level.

REFERENCES

1. Boivin, A., Vendrely, R., and Vendrely, C. L'Acide desoxyribonucleique du noyau cellulaire, dépositaire des caractères hereditaires: Arguments d'ordre analytique. Compt. Rend. Acad. Sci. 226:1961, 1948.
2. Enesco, M., and Leblond, C. P. Increase in cell number as a factor in the growth of the organs of the young male rat, J. Embryol. Exp. Morph. 10:530, 1962.
3. Lapham, L. W. Tetraploid DNA content of Purkinje neurons of human cerebellar cortex, Sci. 159:310, 1968.
4. Epstein, C. J. Cell size, nuclear content, and the development of polyploidy in the mammalian liver. Proc. Nat. Acad. Sci. (U.S.A.) 57:327, 1967.
5. Enesco, M., and Puddy, D. Increase in the number of nuclei and weight in skeletal muscle of rats of various ages, Amer. J. Anat. 114:235, 1964.
6. Winick, M., and Nobel, A. Quantitative changes in DNA, RNA, and protein during prenatal and postnatal growth, Devel. Biol. 12:451, 1965.
7. Holt, L. E., McIntosh, R., and Barnett, H., eds. Pediatrics, 13th ed., New York, Appleton-Century-Crofts, 1962, p. 151.
8. Winick, M. Changes in nucleic acid and protein content of the human brain during growth, Pediat. Res. 2:352, 1968.
9. Mandel, P., Rein, H., Harth-Edel, S., and Mardell, R. Distribution and metabolism of ribonucleic acid in the vertebrate central nervous system, in Comparative Neurochemistry, Richter, D., ed., London, Pergamon Press, 1964, p. 153.
10. Fish, I., and Winick, M. Cellular growth in various regions of the developing rat brain, Pediat. Res. 3:407, 1969.
11. Altman, J. Autoradiographic and histological studies of postnatal neurogenesis. II. A longitudinal investigation of the kinetics, migration and transformation of cells incorporating tritated thymidine in infant rats with special reference to postnatal neurogenesis in some brain regions, J. Comp. Neurol. 128:431, 1966.
12. Altman, J., and Das, G. Autoradiographic and histological studies of

postnatal neurogenesis. I. A longitudinal investigation of the kinetics, migration and transformation of cells incorporating tritiated thymidine in infant rats with special reference to postnatal neurogenesis in some brain regions, J. Comp. Neurol. 126:337, 1966.

13. Winick, M. Nutrition and nerve cell growth, Fed. Proc. 29:1510, 1970.
14. Davison, A. N., and Dobbing, J. The developing brain, in Applied Neurochemistry, Davison, A. N., and Dobbing, J., eds., Oxford, Blackwell Scientific Publications, 1968, p. 253.
15. Manocha, S. L. Malnutrition and Retarded Human Development, Springfield, Ill., Charles C Thomas, 1972.
16. Dobbing, J., and Sands, J. Timing of neuroblast multiplication in developing human brain, Nature 226:639, 1970.
17. Howard, E., Granoff, D. M., and Bujnovsky, P. A. DNA, RNA, and cholesterol increases in cerebrum and cerebellum during development of human fetus, Brain Res. 14:697, 1969.
18. Dobbing, J., and Sands, J. Quantitative growth and development of human brain, Arch. Dis. Child. 48:757, 1973.
19. Winick, M., Rosso, P., and Waterlow, J. Cellular growth of cerebrum, cerebellum, and brain stem in normal and marasmic children, Exptl. Neurol. 26:393, 1970.
20. Duckett, S., and Pearse, A. G. E. The chemo-architectronic patterns of the cerebral cortex of the embryonic and foetal human brain, in Proc. 5th Intl. Cong. of Neuropathology, Excerpta Medica Foundation, Int'l. Cong. Series 100:738, 1966.
21. Duckett, S., and Pearse, A. G. E. Monoamine oxidase cells in the developing human cortex, Rev. Can. Biol. 26:173, 1967.
22. Duckett, S., and Pearse, A. G. E. The cells of Cajal-Retzius in the developing human brain, J. Anat. 102:183, 1968.
23. Duckett, S., and Pearse, A. G. E. Histoenzymology of the developing human spinal cord, Anat. Rec. 163:59, 1969.
24. Nachmansohn, D. Chemical mechanisms of nerve activity, in Modern Trends in Physiology and Biochemistry, Barron, E. S. G., ed., New York, Academic Press, 1952, p. 229.
25. Augustinsson, K. B. Acetylcholine esterase and cholinesterase, in The Enzymes: Chemistry and Mechanism of Action, Vol. 1, Part 1, Sumner, J. B., ed., New York, Academic Press, 1950, p. 443.
26. Im, H. S., Barnes, R. H., Levitsky, D., Krook, L., and Pond, W. C. Postnatal malnutrition and regional cholinesterase activities in brain of pigs, Fed. Proc. 31:697 Abs., 1972.
27. Holstein, I. J., Fish, W. A., and Stokes, W. M. Pathway of cholesterol biosynthesis in the brain of the neonatal rat, J. Lip. Res. 7:364, 1966.
28. Kritchevsky, D., and Holmes, W. L. Occurrence of demosterol in developing rat brain, Biochem. Biophys. Res. Commun. 7:128, 1962.
29. Adams, C. W. M., and Davison, A. N. The occurrence of sterified cholesterol in the developing nervous system, J. Neurochem. 4:282, 1959.
30. Rouser, G., and Yamamoto, A. Lipids, in Handbook of Neurochemistry,

Vol. 1, Chemical Architecture of the Nervous System, Lajtha, A., ed., New York and London, Plenum Press, 1969, p. 121.

31. Evennerholm, L. Distribution and fatty acid composition of phospho-glycerides in normal human brain, J. Lipid Res. 9:570, 1968.

32. Wiegardt, H. The subcellular localization of gangliosides in the brain, J. Neurochem. 14:671, 1967.

33. Dickerson, J. Personal communication.

34. Le Baron, F. Metabolism of myelin constituents, in Handbook of Neuro-chemistry, Vol. 3, Metabolic Reactions in the Nervous System, Lajtha, A., ed., New York and London, Plenum Press, 1970, p. 561.

35. Sperry, W. M. The biochemistry of the brain during early development, in Neurochemistry, Elliott, K. A. C., Page, I. H., and Quastel, J. H., eds., Springfield, Ill., Charles C Thomas, 1962, p. 55.

36. Brante, G. Studies on lipids in nervous system with special reference to quantitative chemical determination and topical distribution, ACTA Physiol. Scand. (Suppl. 63), Stockholm, 18:1, 1949.

37. Cummings, J. N., Goodwin, H., Woodward, E. M., and Curzon, G. Lipids in the brain of infants and children, J. Neurochem. 2:289, 1958.

38. Tingey, A. H. Human brain lipids at various ages in relation to myelina-tion, J. Ment. Sci., London, 102:429, 1956.

39. Howard, E., and Granoff, D. M. Effect of neonatal food restriction in mice on brain growth, DNA and cholesterol and adult delayed response learning, J. Nutr. 95:111, 1968.

40. Altman, J. DNA metabolism and cell proliferation, in Handbook of Neurochemistry, Vol. 2, Structural Neurochemistry, Lajtha, A., ed., New York and London, Plenum Press, 1969, p. 137.

41. Bunge, R. P. Glial cells and the central myelin sheath, Physiol. Rev. 48: 197, 1968.

42. Rosso, P., Hormazabal, J., and Winick, M. Changes in brain weight, cho-lesterol, phospholipid and DNA content in marasmic children, Amer. J. Clin. Nutr. 23:1275, 1970.

43. Porcellati, G. Biochemical processes in brain and nervous tissue, Bibl. "Nutr. Diet." 17:16, Basel, Karger, 1972.

44. Wuzzo, S., Gregory, T., and Gardiner, L. I. Oxygen consumption in brain mitochondria of rats malnourished in utero, J. Nutr. 103:314, 1973.

45. Culley, W. J. Brain energy reserves during early postnatal undernutri-tion, Fed. Proc. 30. No. 2, 459 Abs., 1971.

46. Roberts, E. Formation and utilization of γ-aminobutyric acid in brain, in Progress in Neurobiology. I. Neurochemistry, Vol. 1, Korey, S. R., and Nurnberger, J. I., eds., New York, Hoeber-Harper, 1956, p. 11.

47. Lajtha, A., Berl, S., and Wallsch, H. Amino acid and protein metabolism of the brain. IV. The metabolism of glutamic acid, J. Neurochem. 3:322, 1959.

48. Machiyama, Y., Balazs, R., and Julian, T. Oxidation of glucose through the γ-aminobutyrate pathway in brain, Biochem. J. 96:68, 1965.

49. Tsukada, Y., Shusuka, H., Nagata, Y., and Matsutani, T. Metabolic studies of γ-aminobutric acid in mammalian tissues, in Inhibition in the Nervous System and γ-aminobutyric Acid, Roberts, E., ed., London, Pergamon Press, 1960, p. 163.

50. Baum, D., Brasel, J. A., and Winick, M. Anoxia and DNA content of developing rat brain (in preparation).

51. Neame, D. K. Uptake of histidine, histamine and other imidazole derivatives by brain slices, J. Neurochem. 11:655, 1964.

52. Tsukada, Y., Nagata, Y., Hirano, S., and Matsutani, T. Active transport of amino acids into cerebral cortex slices, J. Neurochem. 10:241, 1963.

53. Guroff, G., Kingl, W., and Udenfriend, S. The uptake of tyrosine by rat brain *in vitro*, J. Biol. Chem. 236:1773, 1961.

54. Wurtman, W. J. Reported at Federation Meetings, Atlantic City, N.J., 1972.

55. Haslam, R. J., and Krebs, H. A. The metabolism of glutamate in homogenates and slices of brain cortex, Biochem. J. 88:566, 1963.

56. Strecker, H. J. Glutamic acid and glutamine, in Metabolism of the Nervous System, Richter, D., ed., London, Pergamon Press, 1957, p. 459.

57. Cravioto, J., Massieu, G., and Izquierdo, J. J. Free amino acids in rat brain during insulinic shock, Proc. Soc. Exp. Biol. Med. 78:856, 1951.

58. Dawson, R. M. C. Studies on the glutamine and glutamic acid content of the rat brain during insulinic hypoglicaemia, Biochem. J. 47:386, 1950.

59. Roff, P. S. de, and Snedeker, E. H. Effect of drugs on amino acid levels in the rat brain and other tissues of rat *in vitro*, Sci. 133:1072, 1961.

60. Aprison, M. H., Davidoff, R. A., and Wermann, R. Glycine. Its metabolic and possible transmitter roles in nervous tissue, in Handbook of Neurochemistry, Vol. III, Lajtha, A., ed., New York, Plenum Press, 1970, p. 381.

61. Bridgers, W. F. The biosynthesis of serine in mouse brain extracts, J. Biol. Chem. 240:4591, 1965.

62. Serini, F., Prinicipi, N., Perletti, L., and Sereni, L. P. Undernutrition and the developing rat brain, Biol. Neonat. 10:254, 1966.

63. Shoemaker, W. J., and Wurtman, R. J. Effect of perinatal undernutrition on the development of the brain catecholamines in the rat, Sci. 171:1017, 1971.

64. Roberts, S., and Morelos, B. S. Regulation of cerebral metabolism of amino acids. IV. Influence of amino acid levels on levels on leucine uptake, utilization and incorporation into protein *in vivo*, J. Neurochem. 12:373, 1965.

65. Harper, A. E. Cited in Mammalian Protein Metabolism, Vol. 2, Munro, H. N., and Allison, J. B., eds., New York, Academic Press, 1964.

66. Clark, H. E. Utilization of essential amino acids by man, in Newer Methods of Nutritional Biochemistry, Vol. II, Albanese, A. A., ed., New York, Academic Press, 1965, p. 123.

67. Richter, D., and Dawson, R. M. C. The ammonia and glutamine content of the brain, J. Biol. Chem. 176:1199, 1948.

68. Lajtha, A., Furst, S., Gerstein, A., and Waelsch, H. Amino acid and protein metabolism of the brain. I. Turnover of free and protein bound lysine in brain and other organs, J. Neurochem. 1:289, 1957.
69. Roberts, S., Zomzely, C. E., and Bondy, S. C. Protein synthesis in the nervous system, in Protein Metabolism of the Nervous System, Lajtha, A., ed., New York, Plenum Press, 1970, p. 3.
70. Porcellati, G., and Curti, B. Proteinase activity of peripheral nerve during Wallerian degeneration, J. Neurochem. 5:277, 1960.
71. Ansell, G. B., and Richter, D. Evidence for a "neutral proteinase" in brain tissue, Biochim. Biophys. Acta 13:92, 1954.
72. Schain, R. J., Carver, M. J., Copenhaver, J. H., and Underhal, N. R. Protein metabolism in the developing brain. Influence of birth and gestational age, Sci. 156:984, 1967.
73. Abdel-Latif, A. A., and Abood, L. G. *In vivo* incorporation of L¹⁴C-serine into phospholipids and proteins of the subcellular fractions of developing rat brain, J. Neurochem. 13:1189, 1966.
74. Oja, S. S. Studies on protein metabolism in developing rat brain, Ann. Acad. Sci. Fenn. 131:1, 1967.
75. Orrego, F., and Lipmann, F. Protein synthesis in brain slices: Effects of electrical stimulation and acidic amino acids, J. Biol. Chem. 242:665, 1967.
76. Wunner, W. H., Bell, J., and Munro, H. N. The effects of feeding with a tryptophane-free amino acid mixture on rat-liver polysome and ribosomal ribonucleic acid, Biochem. J. 101:417, 1966.

Chapter 3 **NUTRITION AND CELLULAR GROWTH OF THE BRAIN**

METHODS FOR PRODUCING EARLY MALNUTRITION

The most common method employed in altering the nutritional status of neonatal rats is to vary the number of pups nursing from a single mother. The normal rat litter consists of from 8 to 12 pups; a nursing group of 10 animals has arbitrarily been considered normal. Malnutrition is imposed by increasing the size of the nursing group to 18 animals, and overnutrition by decreasing the size to 3 animals. But in addition to altering the nutrition, this changes the amount of maternal stimulation available to each pup. More recently, other methods of inducing undernutrition have been employed. Protein restriction in the lactating mother reduces the quantity of milk produced without altering its composition. Allowing the animals to nurse for only a single 8-hour period per day also reduces the quantity of milk consumed. In a combination of these approaches, protein-restricted mothers have been given an increased number of animals to nurse. All of these methods produce a total caloric restriction as well as a restriction in individual nutrients, the most important of which is probably protein. So far, all the methods have had comparable effects on brain growth, and we will therefore examine them together.

In order to produce qualitative changes in maternal milk without altering the quantity, the nursing animal must be artificially fed. This has been done by repeated tube feeding and gastrostomy with continuous infusion of liquid. Both procedures are time-consuming, extremely tedious, and technically difficult. There have not yet been any data compiled on cellular growth of the brain, though Miller has used repeated tube feeding extensively to study protein synthesis in the developing liver.[1]

MALNUTRITION AND BRAIN SIZE

Using the "large and small litter" technique, McCance and Widdowson demonstrated a number of years ago that the growth rate of nursing pups was proportionally slowed down as the number of pups nursing from a single mother was increased.[2] Moreover, they demonstrated that the weight of the brain declined in undernourished animals and rose in overnourished animals. Perhaps their most important finding was that no matter what the state of nutrition after weaning, the undernourished animals never attained normal size and their brains never reached normal adult weight. Other experiments with neonatal pigs confirmed these results. Undernutrition caused profound growth retardation in pigs during the neonatal period and neither body nor brain size ever reached normal adult standards, even when maximum nutritional rehabilitation was attempted.[3] Previous studies had indicated that undernutrition after weaning would retard growth but that nutritional rehabilitation could restore normal body weight and brain weight.[4] What determined whether the animal recovered seemed to be the time at which malnutrition occurred. The earlier the undernutrition, the less likely was recovery. The same difference between early and later growth has been described in dogs.[5] In pups born of malnourished mothers and themselves fed a low protein diet, brain weight relative to the age of the animal was either below or in the lower part of the normal range; this lower average brain size persisted in the adult. When normal bitches were fed a low protein diet during pregnancy and lactation and their offspring were maintained from weaning on a low protein diet, the brain weights of the young pups were below average, but those of five dogs maintained beyond 90 days of age fell within the lower part of the normal range. In other animals born of and suckled by well-fed mothers and first put on deficient diets at age 6 to 7 weeks, the brains were much less severely affected and by 1 year of age were within the normal range for weight.[5] From these studies it would appear that in dogs and pigs, just as in rats, early malnutrition will result in permanent impairment of body and brain growth whereas later malnutrition will produce reversible changes.

MALNUTRITION AND CELLULAR
GROWTH OF THE BRAIN

The studies of normal cellular growth outlined in the preceding chapter suggest a possible explanation for this difference in response between early and late malnutrition. Early organ growth is mainly due to cell division and an increase in the number of cells. Later organ growth is due to hypertrophy with existing cells becoming larger. When the original McCance and Widdowson experiments were repeated and compared with experiments on animals undernourished at two later times during the growing period, it became clear that if malnutrition were imposed during the proliferative phase of growth, the rate of cell division was slowed, and the ultimate number of cells was reduced. Moreover, this change was permanent and could not be reversed once the normal time for cell division had passed. In contrast, undernutrition imposed during the period of hypertrophy will curtail the cellular enlargement, but on subsequent rehabilitation the cells will regain their normal size. These experiments demonstrated that total brain cell number could be permanently reduced by undernourishing the rat during the first 21 days of life; no matter what feeding regimen was attempted thereafter this reduction in cell number persisted.[6]

If the reduction in brain size in the animals reared in litters of 18 was due to a reduced number of cells, what about the animals reared in litters of 3? In this experiment the overnourished animals clearly had an increased number of brain cells when compared with animals nursed in normal-size litters. Subsequent experiments demonstrated that the rate of cell division can actually be manipulated in either direction by changing the state of nutrition during the proliferative phase. Undernutrition for the first 9 days of life produces a deficit in brain cell number which can be entirely overcome by overnutrition during the next 12 days[7] (Fig. 3-1 summarizes the results of these various manipulations). It should be noted, however, that we cannot differentiate one cell type from another using these methods. It is quite possible that the deficit is made up by the proliferation of a different type of cell than was inhibited during the earlier restriction.

These findings have helped to establish a principle of considerable biological importance: that the number of cells present in any organ at

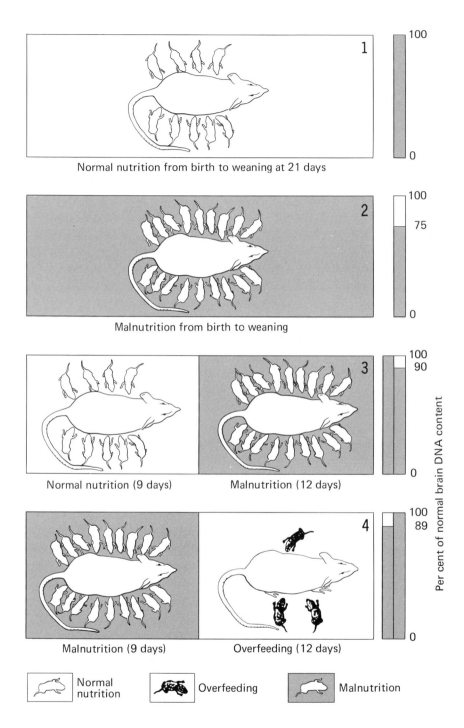

Normal nutrition from birth to weaning at 21 days

Malnutrition from birth to weaning

Normal nutrition (9 days)   Malnutrition (12 days)

Malnutrition (9 days)   Overfeeding (12 days)

Normal nutrition   Overfeeding   Malnutrition

Per cent of normal brain DNA content

Fig. 3.1. Methods of altering nutritional status during the suckling period

maturity is only partially under genetic control. Environmental variables during the proliferative phase of cellular growth also have a part in determining the ultimate number of cells, not by altering the time during which cells can divide but rather by altering the rate at which cell division occurs during the time prescribed by the genetic make-up of the animal. Thus malnutrition slows the rate of cell division but cells do continue to divide for the same period of time in the malnourished animal as in the normal animal.

MALNUTRITION AND MYELINATION

In rats, malnutrition during the first three weeks of life has been shown to interfere with the synthesis of lipids.[8, 9, 10] Total brain cholesterol and cholesterol concentration are reduced.[3] In pigs malnourished during the first year of life, total brain cholesterol and phospholipid content are markedly reduced and cholesterol concentration is slightly reduced.[3] These changes, both in rats and in pigs, persist even when the animals are rehabilitated for a long time. In addition, it has been demonstrated that the incorporation of sulfatide into the myelin of rat brain is reduced both *in vivo* and *in vitro* by malnutrition during the first 3 weeks of life.[11] Moreover, the activity of galactocerebroside sulfokinase, the enzyme responsible for this incorporation, is also reduced.[11] Although the lower lipid content could be due to a reduction in the number of oligodendroglia, the enzymatic effect suggests that lipid synthesis per cell may also be reduced.

Measuring lipid deposition in order to study myelination gives us two types of data, lipid concentration and total lipid content. The increase in total lipid concentration, which is mainly due to reduction in water content, represents a progressive increase in sheath thickness and has therefore been regarded as a "maturity index." In contrast, the increase in total lipid content represents the growth in length or number of axons and either the elongation of existing myelin sheaths or the laying down of new sheaths. Malnutrition prior to weaning in the rat results not only in fewer or shorter myelin sheaths, as assessed by reduced total brain cholesterol, but also in thinner sheaths, since the concentration of cholesterol is also reduced. In the pig, although the number or length of the sheaths is reduced, the thickness would appear to be nearly normal, since there is very little effect on cholesterol concentration. It has been shown that the concentration of galactosides is markedly reduced in the brains of neonatally malnourished rats and pigs.[12] This would suggest that the number of dendritic arborizations is reduced by malnutrition since, as mentioned in Chapter 2, the concentration of galactosides is an indication of the number of dendritic arborizations. More recently this reduction in the number of dendritic arborizations by malnutrition of neonatal rats has been confirmed by direct histologic observations.

During the past few years studies have been initiated in an attempt to determine whether qualitative changes can be induced in the myelin of the central nervous system as reflected by changes in the concentration of the constituent fatty acids. The dietary manipulation most used is the production of an essential fatty acid deficiency (EFA) in the nursing mother or the weanling pup. When this is done, a number of changes in the composition of brain lipids have been reported. C16:1 and C20:3 fatty acids increase whereas arachidonic acid specifically decreases and a general trend toward increased saturation occurs. These changes, however, appear to be reversible at any time so that restoration of a normal diet will result in a redistribution of fatty acids within the lipid components of the brain and ultimately in a normal fatty acid content of brain lipids.[13]

OTHER EFFECTS OF MALNUTRITION
ON THE GROWING BRAIN

Malnutrition during the first 21 days of life in the rat has been shown to affect the synthesis of certain proteins, the synthesis of certain neurohormones and the activity of certain enzymes involved in both protein and RNA metabolism. There is a reduced synthesis of norepinephrine and serotonin in the brains of malnourished animals.[14] Activity of the enzyme acetylcholesterase increases and in this increase persists into adulthood.[15] These findings have come from studies of whole brain so that it is impossible to know whether or not there are any regionally specific changes in these processes. It is impossible at this time to ascribe functional significance to any of these changes. However, these alterations in neurotransmitter metabolism will, no doubt, eventually be correlated with neurophysiologic changes under their control.

Another area of brain biochemistry which has recently come under scrutiny is the synthesis and deposition of a particular class of proteins, the glycoproteins.[16] These proteins are important because along with gangliosides and certain insoluble proteins they make up a significant portion of axon and nerve ending membranes.[17, 18, 19] Moreover, it is believed by some that because these proteins are capable of rapid configurational change when exposed to changing physiochemical microenvironments, they may be functionally important in nerve cell transmission.[20]

Glycoproteins are deposited during the period of dendritic arborization when the large neuronal network is being formed. Thus, even though their functional significance is still unclear, their content (like the content of gangliosides), would reflect the extent of dendritic arborization and indirectly the number of synapses.

Recent studies strongly suggest that malnutrition imposed in rats shortly after birth will reduce the content of both soluble and insoluble glycoproteins.[16] Moreover, the electrophoretic patterns derived from the brains of these malnourished animals would suggest that qualitative changes in the kinds of glycoproteins present also occur after neonatal malnutrition.[16]

REGIONAL CHANGES INDUCED BY MALNUTRITION

Regional patterns of cellular growth in rat brain are modified by malnutrition during the nursing period.[21] The cerebellum, where the rate of cell division is most rapid, is affected earliest (by 8 days of life) and most markedly.[21] The cerebrum, where cell division occurs at a slower rate, is affected later (at 14 days of life) and less markedly. The effects include a reduced rate of cell division in both areas as well as a reduction in over-all protein synthesis and in the synthesis of various lipids. In addition to these effects on areas of rapid cell division, the increase in DNA content which normally occurs in the hippocampus between the fourteenth and seventeenth days, and which is due to a migration of cells from under the lateral ventricle, is delayed and perhaps even partially prevented[21] (Fig. 3-2). It would thus appear that those regions in which the rate of cell division is highest are affected earliest and most markedly and that cell migration is also curtailed. Whether the reduced cell number in the hippocampus represents interference with the migratory patterns or an inhibition of cell division at the source below the lateral

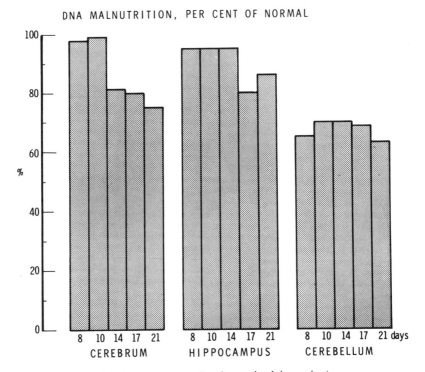

Fig. 3.2. Effect of malnutrition on regional growth of the rat brain

ventricle is not fully known, but data to be discussed shortly strongly suggest that inhibition of cell division accounts at least in part for the reduction.

Regional patterns of lipid synthesis and the effects of malnutrition on these patterns have not been clearly established. The available data, however, suggest that areas where myelination is most rapid are most vulnerable to the effects of early malnutrition.[22] This raises an interesting question that has not yet been investigated. Although the reductions in lipid content and in DNA content are proportional in whole brain, so that the lipid/DNA ratio is unchanged, we cannot interpret this ratio as indicating a normal lipid content per cell. It is conceivable that the reduction in DNA content in a region with little lipid synthesis is matched by a reduction in lipid content in a region where DNA synthesis has already slowed down or stopped. Under these conditions the first region would contain fewer cells but the second region would have reduced lipid content per cell. The actual effect of malnutrition in the area involved in lipid synthesis would be to lower the amount of lipid per cell, but this effect would be masked if both regions were studied together. For this reason it is important that regional studies of the effect of malnutrition on lipid synthesis in the brain be undertaken and correlated with regional studies of DNA synthesis in the same specimens.

As a beginning, it has been shown in rat and pig brain that malnutrition reduces the content of gangliosides in the cerebellum more than that of other lipids, suggesting selective reduction in the quantity of this lipid and hence limitation of dendritic arborization in the cerebellum.[12]

THE EFFECT OF MALNUTRITION ON SPECIFIC TYPES OF CELLS

Three types of studies have examined the various types of cells in the brains of animals malnourished during periods of rapid growth. The first is histologic examination with a variety of special stains. The second is histochemical examination in an attempt to differentiate effects on the developmental patterns of specific enzymes. The third is autoradiography to determine the effects of undernutrition on cell division within particular cell types. Since the same species have not been employed in all of these studies, comparisons are very difficult. Histologic abnormalities have been observed in the central nervous system of rats, pigs, and dogs reared after weaning on protein-deficient diets.[5, 23] The most marked deficits have been observed in dogs. Platt, Heard, and Stewart found abnormalities in the central nervous system in all the protein-calorie deficient animals, whether born of well-fed or malnourished animals. The changes produced were similar in type but varied in degree depending on when the animal was malnourished. Those animals malnourished before birth and during the first 8 to 12 weeks of life showed the most marked alterations. Those malnourished after weaning showed less intense changes.

In pups killed during the phase of acute clinical symptoms, the gray matter showed an excessive concentration of neuroglial nuclei. This increase in neuroglia was not absolute but relative to the number of nerve cells. Thus a disproportion in the relative amount of neurons and glia was observed, producing qualitative as well as quantitative changes in the central nervous system.

Changes within the glial cells themselves were also present. The proportion of neuroglial cells with nuclei of large diameter was increased and cells with elongated vesicular and horseshoe-shaped nuclei were present. Microglial forms, although relatively rare, were more frequent in the congenitally malnourished than in the deficient pups born of normal mothers. Most of the perineuronal (satellite) cells were oligodendroglia but the number of activated astrocytes was also increased. Astrocytic fibers were thicker and more numerous than in control specimens from pups of similar age.

Changes in the nerve cells were also noted. (Fig. 3-3) Many showed varying degrees of chromatolysis, either in their center or periphery or spread throughout the cell. Such cells were often surrounded by oligodendrocytes with indentations of their cell membranes. Actual neuronophagia, however, was observed only rarely. The large motor nerve cells had glial cells closely attached to them, and satellite cells were occasionally so densely packed and enveloped by glial cells that it was difficult to discern their cell nuclei. Some nerve cells had a reduced cytoplasmic con-

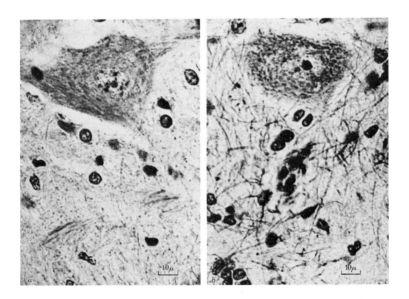

Fig. 3.3. Histologic changes in spinal cord of normal and malnourished puppies. Photomicrographs of nerve cells of the anterior horns of the spinal cords of two puppies aged 3 months. Sections Carnoy-fixed and stained by Mallory's phosphotungstic acid haematoxylin. Left—both pup and mother maintained on a normal diet. Right—mother malnourished during pregnancy and lactation.

tent and if not for the presence of nucleoli could have been mistaken for enlarged astrocytes. Other nerve cells exhibited foamy lattices within the cytoplasm. None of the nerve cells showed an excess of fat, glycogen, or lipofuscin.

Myelination was also curtailed. There was a reduction in the total amount of white matter, especially in those animals malnourished before birth, but no fatty substances or degenerating fibers could be demonstrated. The myelinated fibers of the crossed pyramidal tract had a smaller average area than those of age controls and the deficit was greater at 19 than at 15 weeks of age. This reduction appeared to be at the expense of myelin rather than of the axon itself. The myelin wall was thin in the area adjacent to the anterior fissure. The pyramidal tract in the dog is either very small or absent and the fibers adjacent to the anterior fissure probably represent those of the ventral spinothalamic tract. Stuart and Platt's findings suggest that this important tract was affected by malnutrition.

Once the period of intense clinical signs had passed, few changes remained within the motor nerve cells. However, there was an increased number of neuroglial cells, many with large nuclei, and a fibrous gliosis similar to that seen in a normal 6-year-old dog. The central nervous systems of pups born of malnourished mothers and given good protein diets at weaning were not normal even after two and a half months on these diets; the myelinated fibers had a smaller average diameter, there was an increased concentration of neuroglial cells, the caliber of astrocytic fibers was greater and the "altered" cells were more common than in the tissues of normal animals of similar age.

The changes in the brain stem were of the same type as those described in the spinal cord. The large cells of the reticular formations had a low chromatin content and the Nissl granules were indistinct. This condition also occurred in the third, seventh, and twelfth nerve nuclei, while in many cells of the olivary body and the ascending nucleus of the fifth nerve the amounts of cytoplasm were small and the cell outlines indistinct and uneven.

Since the cells of the cerebral cortex of the normal dog have less chromatin than the spinal cord, the changes were less obvious in the cerebrum. The most marked changes were again a gliosis relative to the number of neurons and some degenerative changes seen in the larger neuronal elements. In cerebellum the individual folia were narrow and the fibrous, granular and molecular layers smaller than in normal controls of equal age. The regular palisade of Purkinje cells was disturbed and in some areas the numbers were reduced and the cells pyknotic. Sections treated to show succinic dehydrogenase activity showed that the cells of the granular layer were less densely packed than in the normal animal. The glutamic dehydrogenase activity of the individual Purkinje cells did not appear to be reduced, but the low concentration of cells possibly led to an over-all deficit. However, the number of Bergmann cells was increased and, as these are sites of strong glutamic dehydrogenase activity, they may have compensated in part for the deficit among the Purkinje cells. Mild degrees of chromatolysis and satellitosis were observed in the dentate nuclei.

These studies of Platt, Heard, and Stewart are the most extensive histological examination of the effects of malnutrition during early life on the brain. They have demonstrated that in puppies malnutrition will have profound effects not only on cellular growth but on myelination and will even cause the death of already existing cells. It should be pointed out, however, that histological studies in certain other species, including the human, have not revealed as marked effects. Whether this is a technical problem or whether the dog is more susceptible to neonatal malnutrition is at present not clear.

In pigs milder changes have been demonstrated with severe undernutrition early in life, especially in the cortex itself.[5] Neurons in the gray matter are reduced in number and appear swollen. More recently, histological changes have been described in the brains of rats subjected to early malnutrition.[24] The appearance of a variety of enzymes demonstrable by special staining techniques is delayed, and the ultimate quantity obtained is reduced. In a very recent study the effect of malnutrition and subsequent rehabilitation on the somatosensory area of the cerebral cortex was studied in young rats. Quantitative differential cell counts indicated that undernutrition during either gestation or lactation reduced non-neuronal components to a greater extent than neurons. Partial recovery with rehabilitation was mainly due to an increase in the number of glial and endothelial cells of the cerebral cortex. The earlier the malnutrition the more marked the effects.[25]

In a study of squirrel monkeys born of protein-restricted mothers defects in the fetal brain and spinal cord were found. Neuronal elements were reduced, many neurons appeared pyknotic, and there was evidence of gliosis. Moreover, special staining techniques revealed a marked reduction in the activity of certain enzymes in both neurons and glia.[26]

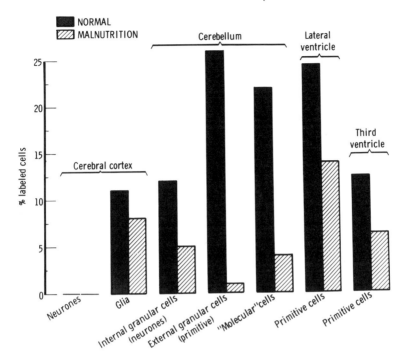

Fig. 3.4. Effect of malnutrition on individual cell types in rat brain

Autoradiographic studies in our laboratory indicate that in neonatal rats malnourished for the first 10 days of life, only glial cell division is inhibited in the cerebrum since neuronal cell division ceases before birth.[27] In cerebellum, the rate of cell division of external granular cells, internal granular cells, and molecular cells is reduced. In addition, the rate of cell division in neurons under both the third and lateral ventricles is decreased. This reduction in neurons under the lateral ventricle explains, at least in part, the reduced DNA content in the hippocampus 5 days later, since these are the cells that are destined to migrate into the hippocampus (Fig. 3-4).

MALNUTRITION AND CELLULAR GROWTH OF PERIPHERAL NERVES

All of the work outlined thus far has been concerned with changes induced in the developing central nervous system. Recently there have been studies of the effect of early malnutrition on the development of peripheral nerves in young rats.[28] Careful analysis has revealed that undernutrition initiated early in life reduces the caliber of nerve fibers in the sciatic nerve and its roots. This reduction is most marked in the thicker fibers. Myelin deposition is also impaired in the ventral and dorsal root fibers and in the fibers of other peripheral nerves such as the optic nerve. The quantitative effect of early malnutrition varies with the particular nerve being examined. In the ventral root fibers, myelin deposition is curtailed more than axonal expansion. In the dorsal root fibers the reduction in myelination and radial axonal growth is proportional. In the optic nerve the effect on axonal growth is greater than on myelination.

Rehabilitation also will produce different changes depending on the nerve or root studied. The reduction of the caliber and reduced myelin content in the dorsal root fibers persists even after a long period of nutritional rehabilitation. In the ventral root all the changes were completely reversible. In both the sciatic and optic nerves partial recovery took place. These studies demonstrate that malnutrition early in life can induce changes in peripheral nerves similar to those described in the central nervous system. Some of the changes are reversible whereas others are not. Certain nerves and roots are more susceptible than others. This work is only beginning but could yield important findings which might help in our understanding of some of the deficits produced by early malnutrition.

POSSIBLE MECHANISMS BY WHICH MALNUTRITION MAY AFFECT CELLULAR GROWTH OF THE BRAIN

How does malnutrition exert its effect on cell division? The elucidation of these mechanisms is one of the most important future directions for scientists interested in malnutrition and brain development. During the past few years a number of laboratories have begun to address themselves to this problem.

Since it has been known for a long time that various hormones, particularly growth hormone and thyroid hormone, are very important in the control of normal growth, there has been a good deal of speculation that malnutrition exerts its effects on growth indirectly by reducing the amount or availability of one or both of these hormones. This concept of an indirect effect of malnutrition exerted primarily through the endocrine system has been supported by some data while other data have failed to support the concept. For example, certain workers have observed increased growth in malnourished animals injected with growth hormone.[29] Others have not.[30] In neonatally undernourished rats, reduced thyroid hormone in the circulation has been reported as well as a reduced oxygen consumption in brain, a known consequence of thyroid deficiency.[31] Circulating growth hormone has been reported to be reduced in human infants with marasmus and their growth rate increased if treated with growth hormone.[32] By contrast, in the case of kwashiorkor, growth hormone levels are elevated and yet growth failure is prominent.[33] Recent data have begun to shed some light on the role of hormones in the growth retardation produced by early malnutrition.

In rats, hypothyroidism reduces the rate of cell division in brain but extends the time during which cells divide from 21 days to about 35 days. The ultimate number of cells achieved is actually greater than in normal animals. By contrast hyperthyroidism produces the reverse. The rate of cell division is increased but the time is shortened and the ultimate number of cells is fewer.[34] As we have seen, the effects of a change in nutritional status during early life are always on the rate of cell division. The time during which cells divide is never altered. In rat brain, cell division ceases at 21 days regardless of how the animal is fed. We can see, therefore, that there is a fundamental difference between the action or lack of action of thyroid hormone and that of malnutrition. This difference is highlighted if one examines the activity of DNA polymerase (an enzyme involved in DNA synthesis) in hypothyroidism and in malnutrition. Hypothyroid animals show lower activity during the early hyperplastic phase of brain growth. However, activity remains elevated beyond the period of time when it drops to low levels in normal brain. By contrast, in malnourished animals, activity drops to these low (adult) levels at the normal time[34] (Fig. 3-5).

These data clearly demonstrate that the effects of early malnutrition are not manifesting themselves, at a cellular level, by reducing either the secretion or the availability of thyroid hormone.

The role of pituitary growth hormone in producing the effects of malnutrition is less clearly defined. Growth hormone deficiency reduces the rate of cell division without altering the time that cells divide. In this respect, then, its effect is similar to that of undernutrition. In growth hormone deficiency, however, this reduction in the rate of cell division in all organs does not take place until the middle part of neonatal life. For ex-

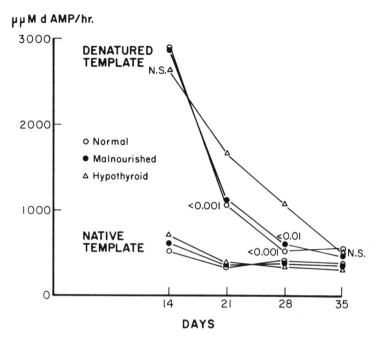

μμM d AMP/hr.

Fig. 3.5. The effect of hypothyroidism and malnutrition on DNA polymerase activity in rat brain

ample, in mice genetically devoid of growth hormone, organ growth and the rate of cell division in the various organs is normal during the first 10 days of life[35] (Fig. 3-6). Thus early hyperplastic growth both prenatally and during early neonatal life is not under the control of growth hormone, yet undernutrition will reduce the rate of cell division during this period of life. These data suggest that at least during gestation and early lactation, the period when brain changes are most marked, malnutrition exerts its effects independent of growth hormone. The possibility still exists, however, that one of the effects of malnutrition is to inhibit the secretion of growth hormone and therefore to limit its availability when it is needed. Assuming that this were so, it would seem most logical that this effect is in addition to the primary effect of malnutrition on cellular growth, which continues to be the same both before and after growth hormone becomes important. Recent data would support this interpretation. "Overnutrition" increases the rate of protein synthesis in pituitary dwarf mice during the time that cell division has stopped.[36] Malnutrition reduces the activity of the enzyme serine dehydrogenase in

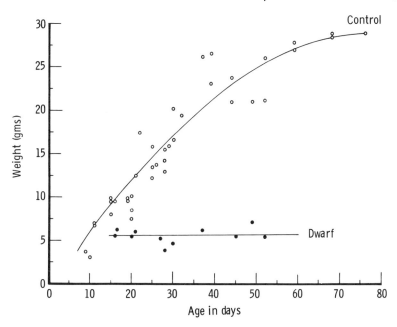

Fig. 3.6. Growth of hypopituitary dwarf mice. In comparison to normal littermates, the dwarf mice demonstrate considerable growth retardation first noted at 10 to 12 days of age. Prior to that time body weight measurements reveal no differences from control values.

growing liver. Hypophysectomy has no effect.[37] When treated with growth hormone malnourished animals show little or no increase in DNA synthesis.[38] Finally, animals re-fed after malnutrition show a return to normal in cellular growth much more rapidly than do hypophysectomized rats treated with growth hormone. Thus the data at present would indicate that malnutrition does not act by reducing the availability or secretion of growth hormone in early hyperplastic growth and that, even during later growth, malnutrition does not act solely through this mechanism. What then is the primary mechanism by which undernutrition affects cellular growth?

Figure 3-7 is an oversimplified scheme depicting some of the events taking place during cellular growth and cell division. Amino acids from the general body pool are supplied directly for protein synthesis and for the synthesis of nucleotides which then enter the general body nucleotide pool. The nucleotides are then utilized for either DNA or RNA synthesis. Newly formed DNA is quite stable, whereas the newly formed RNA

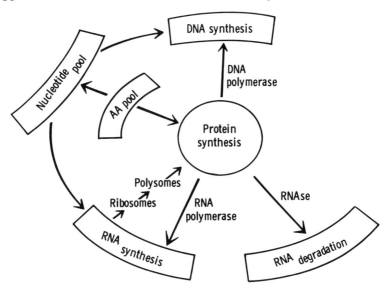

Fig. 3.7. Various aspects of cell biochemistry during normal growth

turns over and the rate of synthesis is in equilibrium with the rate of degradation. A number of enzymes are involved in all of these processes; their activity depends, in part at least, on the quantitative and qualitative nature of protein synthesis. Thus the availability of amino acids will affect both nucleic acid and protein synthesis, and the amount and quality of the protein synthesized will in turn affect the synthesis of nucleic acids. To complete the cycle, since RNA is an essential element in protein synthesis, changes in the quantity and quality of RNA will also affect the quantity and quality of the protein synthesized.

Where in this cycle does protein-calorie malnutrition exert its effect? Although the data are not complete, they certainly point to the fact that limitation of protein in the diet will decrease the availability of amino acids for protein synthesis. The work of Munro[39] and more recently that of Miller[40] has demonstrated reduced protein synthesis both *in vivo* and *in vitro* when either protein or amino acids in the diet are limited. Further, Munro has suggested that although any amino acid may be limiting under experimental conditions, tryptophane appears to be the limiting amino acid in most physiological situations.[39] Thus although definitive proof awaits measurement of amino acid pool size and tracking of amino acid pathways under conditions of protein-calorie malnutrition, the evidence at present strongly suggests that the amino acid pool size is reduced. How is this reduced quantity of amino acid distributed? Amino acids for building blocks of protein are less available as shown by the decreased incorporation of labeled amino acids into total protein. In contrast, there is some evidence which suggests that amino acids are preferentially converted to nucleotides. For example, total nucleotide pool size in brains of neonatally malnourished animals is unaffected. However incorporation of labeled orotic acid into the nucleotide pool is significantly increased, and preliminary data suggest that incorporation of labeled amino acids into the nucleotide pool is also increased.[41] We may postulate then that the synthesis of nucleotides is increased in brains of neonatally malnourished rats. If the nucleotide pool size does not change in brain or actually decreases in liver, where are these nucleotides being distributed? Incorporation of labeled nucleotides into DNA is markedly reduced in the brains of malnourished animals, demonstrating that there is a decreased distribution into DNA synthesis. In contrast, incorporation of labeled precursor into RNA is markedly increased in brains of neonatally malnourished animals.[41] Thus the rate of DNA synthesis is reduced, whereas the rate of RNA synthesis is increased in neonatal protein-calorie restriction. One effect, then, of early malnutrition is a redistribution of available nucleotides. How is this redistribution controlled? What are the mechanisms involved in the decreased DNA synthesis and how can we explain an increase in RNA synthesis in the face of descriptive data which conclusively demonstrate a reduced RNA content per cell?

We can answer the second question by examining the rate of RNA degradation after early malnutrition. There is a marked increase in the rate of decay of previously labeled RNA in liver of malnourished rats and in brain there is a drop in the RNA/DNA ratio at a time when RNA synthesis is increased.[42] Thus although the rate of RNA synthesis is increased the rate of degradation must also be increased. This latter increase is presumably greater than the former, resulting in a net loss of RNA which explains the drop in the RNA/DNA ratio or RNA content per cell.

At this point, we may summarize the effects of early malnutrition on some of the synthetic and degradative pathways involved in cellular growth. Incorporation of amino acids into total protein is reduced as is net protein synthesis. Incorporation of labeled precursors into the nucleotide pool is increased in the face of an unchanging or dropping total nucleotide pool size. Incorporation of nucleotides into DNA is decreased as is net DNA synthesis. Incorporation of nucleotides into RNA is increased, suggesting an increased rate of RNA synthesis in the face of a decrease in cellular RNA content. The rate of RNA degradation is markedly increased.

In an attempt to explore some of the mechanisms by which these dynamic changes occur, the activity of certain of the enzymes involved in the regulation of the steps just described has been measured. DNA polymerase is an enzyme involved in the terminal phase of DNA synthesis. In a number of nonphysiological situations the activity of this enzyme has been shown to increase under conditions which stimulate DNA synthesis.[43, 44] Moreover, the increase has been shown to precede the increase in DNA synthesis.[44] Recent experiments in our laboratory have demonstrated that the response to unilateral nephrectomy in the opposite kidney is hyperplastic in infant rats and hypertrophic in adult rats.[45] This hyperplastic response is preceded by a burst of DNA polymerase activity in the remaining kidney of the infant animal whereas the polymerase response in the adult is much smaller.[44]

More recently it has been shown that activity of this enzyme in liver of growing rats is in part under the control of pituitary growth hormone. Hypophysectomy reduces enzyme activity and growth hormone replacement elevates the activity before any increase in DNA synthesis can be demonstrated[38] (Fig. 3-8).

In brain we have demonstrated that the activity of DNA polymerase parallels the rate of cell division during normal growth[46] and that this parallel relationship holds when various brain regions are studied[49] (Fig. 3-9). These data demonstrate that the activity of this enzyme is an excellent indicator of the rate of cell division and suggest that during normal growth DNA polymerase may play a role in regulating the rate of DNA synthesis. Neonatal malnutrition will reduce the activity of this enzyme in rat liver. Recently, Jasper and Brasel have demonstrated that when malnourished animals are re-fed during the hyperplastic phase of growth, the activity of DNA polymerase returns to normal levels within 12 hours. By 24 hours activity is 150% of normal. DNA synthesis as measured either by C^{14} thymidine incorporation into DNA or by increases in total DNA content does not increase for at least 48 hours[48] (Fig. 3-10). These data clearly demonstrate an increase in activity of DNA polymerase *before* any demonstrable increase in DNA synthesis and suggest that increased levels in the activity of this enzyme stimulates DNA synthesis

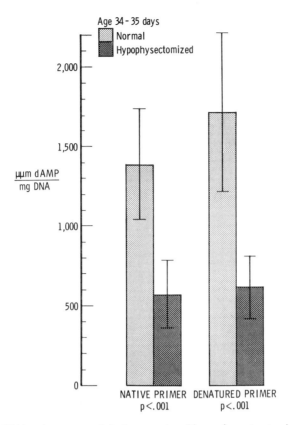

Fig. 3.8.   DNA polymerase activity in normal and hypophysectomized rat kidney

rather than the reverse. These findings reinforce other data, some of which were cited previously, in suggesting that DNA polymerase activity during both normal and abnormal growth plays a role in regulating the rate of cell division.

Thus the evidence at this stage suggests that one way by which early malnutrition may curtail the rate of DNA synthesis and perhaps indirectly regulate the distribution of available nucleotides is by reducing the activity of DNA polymerase.

While we have not investigated the enzymes involved in RNA synthesis, others have begun such investigations. Metcoff and co-workers have demonstrated an increase in RNA polymerase activity in leukocytes of undernourished children and in placentas from mothers who were malnourished and whose infants demonstrated intrauterine growth failure.[49]

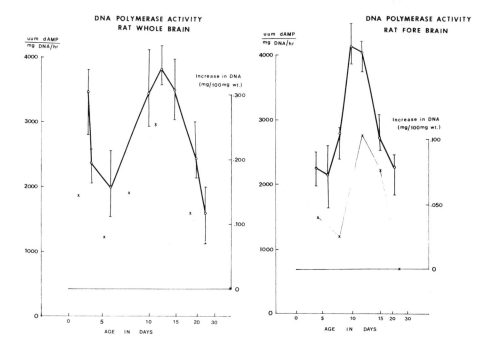

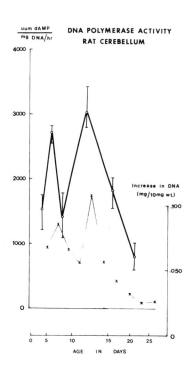

Fig. 3.9. DNA polymerase activity in normal rat brain during development. Polymerase activity is shown by open circles, with brackets representing range of data and *not* SDs. Rate of increase in DNA is shown by closed circles. DNA rate curve parallels curve for enzyme activity.

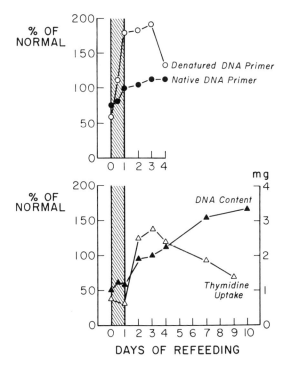

Fig. 3.10.   Effects of refeeding on liver DNA content. (▲—▲), radiothymidine uptake (△—△), and DNA polymerase activity (●—● native DNA template, O—O de-
natured DNA template).

Suggestive as these data may be, experiments demonstrating an elevation
in the activity of RNA polymerase in tissues exposed to neonatal malnutrition, and correlating this increased activity with an increase in the
rate of RNA synthesis, are lacking.

The degradative phase of RNA metabolism is of particular interest
since it is the increased rate of degradation which accounts for the net
loss of RNA per cell. The enzyme alkaline RNase has been presumed to
be involved in RNA catabolism. Available data suggest that under most
circumstances activity of this enzyme is inversely related to cellular RNA
content.[50] We have therefore undertaken a series of investigations designed to explore the role of this enzyme during normal growth and the
alterations that may occur in early malnutrition. During normal brain development the activity of this enzyme per cell increases, but this increase
is exactly proportional to the increase in cellular RNA content, keeping

the relationship between enzyme and substrate constant throughout development. Total activity of alkaline RNase increases per milligram of DNA (per cell) throughout development except for a drop at birth and again at 17 days of age. By contrast specific activity (activity per mg of protein) declines during development. When activity is expressed per milligram of RNA (per mg of substrate), there is no change during development[51] (Fig. 3-11). These data emphasize the importance of the mode of expression of enzyme activity and point out clearly that interpretation of changes in such activity may depend a great deal on the reference point employed. By using these three reference points, a clearer picture can be developed. Activity per cell increases during brain development; this increase is less than the increase in other cellular proteins and hence the specific activity drops. However, the increased activity per cell is directly proportional to the increase in RNA content per cell which occurs during development, and therefore the activity per milligram of RNA does not change. This constant relationship between RNase activity and RNA content under circumstances where both are changing again suggests a role for this enzyme in the regulation of RNA

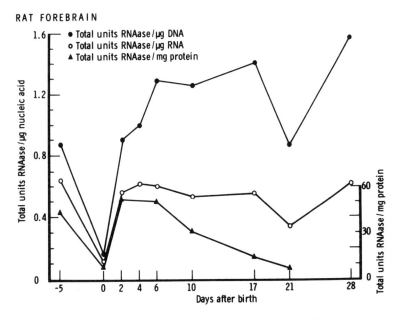

Fig. 3.11. Activity of free alkaline ribonuclease during normal development in rat forebrain

metabolism. In the above studies only total cellular alkaline RNase activity was studied because of initial findings of very small amounts of free activity (non-inhibitor bound) in the nuclear and cytoplasmic fractions.

In other tissues, however, alkaline RNase is active intranuclearly, as well as in the cytoplasm, and is present as both bound and free enzyme.[52] Preliminary data suggest that the nuclear activity is in some manner related to the rate of RNA synthesis within the nucleus, whereas the cytoplasmic enzyme is involved in the regulation of RNA catabolism in the cytoplasm. For example, if one examines the activity of cytoplasmic RNase in three different adult tissues which catabolize RNA at three different rates, a direct correlation between enzyme activity and rate of catabolism is immediately apparent. The most rapid rate of RNA degradation occurs in kidney, with liver and brain following in descending order. The highest activity of RNase per cell also occurs in kidney, with liver and brain following respectively. Moreover, the differences in enzyme activity are directly proportional to the differences in catabolic rate.[53]

These data strongly suggest that alkaline RNase must play a role in the regulation of RNA metabolism and, indirectly, protein synthesis by influencing the rate of RNA catabolism. Since, as previously pointed out, RNA catabolism is increased in brains of animals exposed to early malnutrition, the effect of such malnutrition on the activity of alkaline RNase has been studied. Malnutrition imposed at birth will elevate the activity of this enzyme in rat brain[54] (Fig. 3-12). This elevation progressively increases as the duration of malnutrition increases, so that increased activity is present regardless of whether the data are expressed per milligram of DNA, per milligram of protein, or per milligram of RNA. Thus neonatal malnutrition selectively elevates the activity of this enzyme in the face of a decrease in over-all protein synthesis and a fall in tissue RNA content.

At this point let me summarize what is known about the effects of early malnutrition on cellular growth of the brain and present a hypothesis as to how malnutrition affects the regulatory mechanisms involved in the control of cellular growth (Fig. 3-13). Malnutrition during proliferative growth will curtail net protein, RNA, and DNA synthesis and result in an organ with a reduced number of cells. It would appear that any cell type in a region where cells are dividing is vulnerable to the effects of nutritional deprivation. Early malnutrition limits the availability of amino acids for incorporation into protein, thereby reducing the rate of protein synthesis. By contrast, an increased flow of amino acids enters the nu-

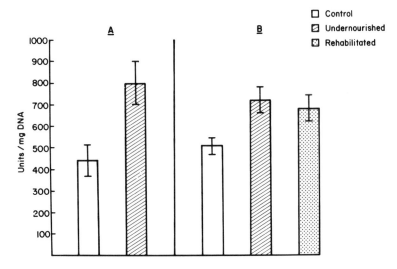

Fig. 3.12.   The effect of undernutrition on free ribonuclease activity in rat forebrain (A) at 14 days of age, (B) at 21 days of age. Values 3% mean + S.E. of five animals

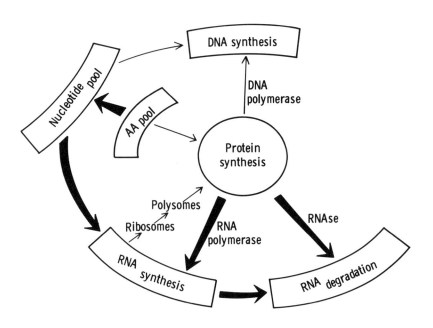

Fig. 3.13.   Various aspects of cell biochemistry during malnutrition

cleotide pool; this increased flow presumably limits even further the availability of these amino acids for protein synthesis. Nucleotides are removed from the pool much more slowly along the pathway to DNA synthesis, since the synthesis of DNA is occurring at a much slower rate than normal. This reduced rate of DNA synthesis is in part at least a consequence of the reduced activity of certain enzymes involved in that synthesis, for example DNA polymerase. By contrast, nucleotides are removed much more quickly along the pathway to RNA synthesis, since synthesis of RNA is more rapid than normal. This results in either a depletion in the size of the nucleotide pool, as occurs in liver, or a maintenance of normal amounts, as occurs in brain. However, regardless of the effect on pool size, the distribution from the pool has been altered by early undernutrition. The increase in RNA synthesis may direct alterations in protein synthesis which result in selective elevations in certain proteins, for example RNA polymerase and alkaline RNase. The increased RNA polymerase activity may further stimulate the enhanced RNA synthesis, whereas the increased activity of alkaline RNase may initiate the increased rate of RNA degradation which has been demonstrated. This increased catabolic phase may in turn be responsible for the shift in polysome pattern described by Munro, and through this mechanism may contribute even further to the selective reduction in protein synthesis.

MALNUTRITION AND CELLULAR GROWTH
OF THE HUMAN BRAIN

Studies of the effects of malnutrition on cellular growth of the human brain have been limited. In marasmic infants who died of malnutrition during the first year of life, wet weight, dry weight, total protein, total RNA, total cholesterol, total phospholipid, and total DNA content are proportionally reduced.[55, 56] Thus, the rate of DNA synthesis is slowed and cell division is curtailed, reducing the number of cells. Since the reduction in the other elements is proportional to the reduction in DNA content, the ratios are unchanged and the size of cells as well as the lipid or RNA content of the individual cell is not altered (Fig. 3-14). Again it should be emphasized that we are describing "average" cells and it is quite possible that certain cells, that is, those in which lipid is being actively deposited, are affected differently. If the malnutrition persists be-

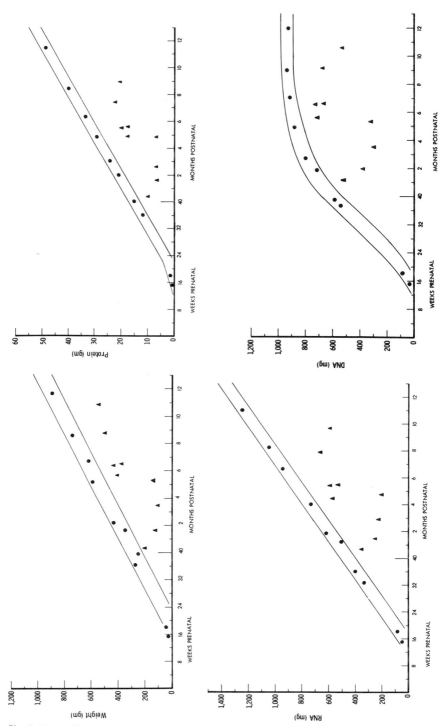

Fig. 3.14. Cellular growth in the brains of normal and malnourished children. Lines indicate normal range for U.S. population. ● indicates normal Chilean children. ▲ indicates Chilean children who died of severe malnutrition during first year of life.

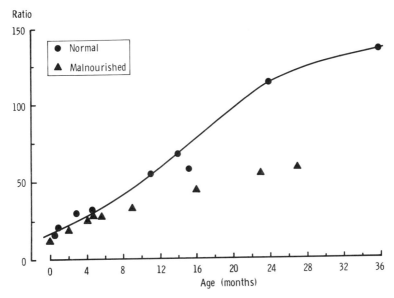

Fig. 3.15. Lipid-DNA ratio in normal and malnourished children at different ages

yond about 8 months of age, not only the number of cells but also their size is reduced. In addition, the lipid per cell is also reduced (Fig. 3-15).

Thus in the human brain there is a type of response to malnutrition similar to that which has been described in lower animals. During proliferative growth cell division is curtailed; during hypertrophic growth the normal enlargement of cells is prevented. From our discussion of normal lipid metabolism in brain in the previous chapter we can interpret the effects of malnutrition on the human brain as affecting myelination in a manner more analogous to the effects on pig than to those on the rat brain. Total cholesterol or phospholipid content is reduced; hence the number or length of myelin sheaths is reduced. But because both phospholipid and cholesterol concentration are unaffected, the thickness of those myelin sheaths that are present is unaffected (Fig. 3-16). One could then argue that the major effect of malnutrition is to interfere with cellular growth. During the first 8 months of life this interference reduces the number of glia, specifically oligodendroglia, and myelination is proportionally reduced. Continued malnutrition reduces cell size. In neurons this would probably be associated with a reduction in the number or

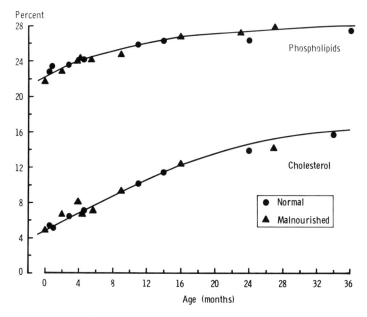

Fig. 3.16. Cholesterol and phospholipid concentration per 100 g. dry tissue in normal and malnourished children at different ages

length of processes, and myelination would be proportionally curtailed. However, the deposition of myelin around those processes which are present and which do grow proceeds normally. Note that this interpretation is based on limited observations.

Recently it has been shown that galactoside *concentration* is reduced in the brains of human infants who died of severe malnutrition.[57] This would indicate that, as in rats and pigs, early undernutrition will selectively reduce the concentration of certain gangliosides in the human brain. If ganglioside concentration reflects the number of dendritic arborizations, then the process of dendritic branching may be retarded by early undernutrition.

Malnutrition in the human reduces the rate of cell division in all three areas of the brain studied to date: cerebrum, cerebellum, and brain stem (Fig. 3-17). As in experimental animals malnutrition will thus curtail cell division in any brain region undergoing hyperplastic growth.

It now seems clear that early postnatal malnutrition will affect both cell division and myelination in the developing rat and human brain. In

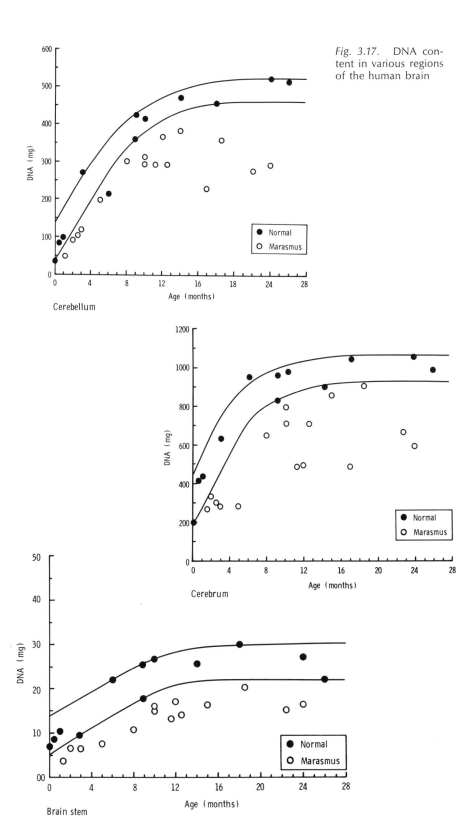

Fig. 3.17. DNA content in various regions of the human brain

both species it would appear that the vulnerable periods coincide with the maximum rate of synthesis of DNA and of myelin. All brain regions seem to be vulnerable, but the timing of their vulnerability will vary, again depending on the maximum rate of synthesis in the particular region. All cell types so far studied are affected if they are dividing at the time the undernutrition occurs. Finally, there is a selective reduction in the number of dendritic arborizations in the rat, pig, and human brain subjected to early undernutrition. In the rat, recovery appears to be possible only if the nutritional status is changed during these vulnerable periods. In the human, although we cannot prove it, we must presume that the same is true.

REFERENCES

1. Miller, S. A. Protein metabolism during growth and development, in Mammalian Protein Metabolism, Vol. 3, Munro, H. N., ed., New York, Academic Press, 1969, p. 189.
2. Widdowson, E. M., and McCance, R. A. Some effects of accelerating growth. I. General somatic development, Proc. Roy. Soc., London 152: 88, 1960.
3. Dickerson, J. W. T., Dobbing, J., and McCance, R. A. The effect of undernutrition on the postnatal development of the brain and cord in pigs, Proc. Roy. Soc., London, B. 166:396, 1966–67.
4. Jackson, C. M., and Steward, C. A. The effects of inanition in the young upon the ultimate size of the body and of the various organs in the albino rat, J. Exptl. Zool. 30:97, 1920.
5. Platt, B. S. Proteins in nutrition, Proc. Roy. Soc., London, 156:337, 1962.
6. Winick, M., and Noble, A. Cellular response in rats during malnutrition at various ages, J. Nutr. 89:300, 1966.
7. Winick, M., Fish, I., and Rosso, P. Cellular recovery in rat tissues after a brief period of neonatal malnutrition, J. Nutr. 95:623, 1968.
8. Davison, A. N., and Dobbing, J. The developing brain, in Applied Neurochemistry, Davison, A. N., and Dobbing, J. eds., Oxford, Blackwell Scientific Publications, 1968, p. 253.
9. Culley, W. J., and Lineberger, R. Effect of undernutrition on the size and composition of the rat brain, J. Nutr. 96:375, 1968.
10. Davison, A. N., and Dobbing, J. Myelination as a vulnerable period in brain development, Brit. Med. Bull. 22:40, 1966.
11. Chase, H. P., Dorsey, J., and McKhann, G. M. The effect of malnutrition on the synthesis of a myelin lipid, Pediatrics 40:551, 1967.
12. Dickerson, J. W. T. Personal communication.

13. Galli, C. Dietary lipids in brain development, in Dietary Lipids in Post-natal Development, Galli, C., Jacini, C., and Pecile, A., eds. New York, Raven Press, 1973, p. 191.

14. Shoemaker, W. J., and Wurtman, R. J. Effect of perinatal undernutrition on the development of the brain catecholamines in the rat, Science 171: 1017, 1971.

15. Im, H. S., Barnes, R. H., Levitsky, D., Krook, L., and Pond, W. C. Postnatal malnutrition and regional cholinesterase activities in brain of pigs, Fed. Proc. 31:697 Abs., 1972.

16. Di Benedetta, C., and Cioffi, L. A. Early malnutrition, brain glycoproteins and behavior in rats, Bibl. Nutr. Diet. 17:68, 1972.

17. Rambourg, A., and Leblond, C. P. Electron microscopic observations on the carbohydrate-rich cell coat present at the surfaces of cells in the rat, J. Cell Biol. 32:27, 1967.

18. Pease, D. C. Polysaccharides associated with the exterior surface of epithelial cells: kidney, intestine, brain, J. Ultrastruct. Res. 15:555, 1966.

19. Brunngraber, E. G., Dekirmenjian, H., and Brown, B. D. The distribution of protein-bound N-acetylneuraminic acid in subcellular fractions of rat brain, Biochem. J. 103:73, 1968.

20. Schmitt, F. O., and Davison, P. F. Brain and nerve proteins. Functional correlates. Proteins and biolectric functions, Neurosci. Res. Progr. Bull. 3:1, 1965.

21. Fish, I., and Winick, M. The effects of malnutrition on regional growth of the developing rat brain, Exptl. Neurol. 25:534, 1969.

22. Culley, W. J. Reported at Federation Meetings, Atlantic City, 1971.

23. Platt, B. S., Heard, C. R. C., and Stewart, R. J. C. Experimental protein calorie deficiency, in Mammalian Protein Metabolism, Vol. 2, Munro, H. R., and Allison, J. B., eds., New York, Academic Press, 1964, p. 445.

24. Zeman, F. J. Reported at Federation Meetings, Atlantic City, N.J., 1972.

25. Zeman, F. J. Reported at Federation Meetings, Atlantic City, N.J., 1973.

26. Manocha, S. L. Cited in Malnutrition and Retarded Human Development, Springfield, Ill., Charles C Thomas, 1972.

27. Winick, M. Cellular growth in intrauterine malnutrition, Pediat. Cl. No. Amer. 17:69, 1970.

28. Sima, A. Cited in Studies on Calibre Growth of Nerve Fibres and Perineural Permeability in Normal, Undernourished, and Rehabilitated Rats, Goteborg, Sweden, Neuropathological Laboratory, Institute of Pathology, University of Goteborg, 1974.

29. Zamenhof, S., Van Marthens, E., and Grauel, L. Prenatal cerebral development: Effect of restricted diet, reversal by growth hormone, Science 174:954, 1971.

30. Jasper, H., and Brasel, J. A. Unpublished observations.

31. Muzzo, S., Gregory, T., and Gardner, L. I. Oxygen consumption by brain mitochondria of rats malnourished in utero, J. Nutr. 103:314, 1973.

32. Monckeberg, F., Donoso, G., Oxman, S., Pak, N., and Meneghello, J.

Human growth hormone in infant malnutrition, Pediatrics 31:58, 1963.
33. Pimstone, B. L., Becker, D. J., and Hansen, J. D. L. Human growth hormone and sulphation factor in protein-calorie malnutrition, in Endocrine Aspects of Malnutrition, Kroc Foundation Symposium No. 1, Gardner, L. I., and Amacher, P., eds., Santa Ynez, Calif., Kroc Foundation, 1973, p. 73.
34. Muzzo, S., and Brasel, J. A. Neonatal hypothyroidism and DNA synthesis in rat cerebellum, presented at the 55th Annual Meeting of the Endocrine Society, June 1973.
35. Winick, M., and Grant, P. Cellular growth in the organs of the hypo-pituitary dwarf mouse, Endocr. 83:544, 1968.
36. Winick, M. Cellular response with increased feeding in pituitary dwarf mice, J. Nutr. 94:121, 1968.
37. Rosso, P. Personal communication.
38. Jasper, H., and Brasel, J. A. The effects of growth hormone on DNA polymerase activity in the liver of normal and hypophysectomized rats, Endocr. 92:194, 1973.
39. Munro, H. N. Reported at Federation Meetings, Atlantic City, N.J., 1970.
40. Miller, S. A. Protein metabolism during growth and development, in Mammalian Protein Metabolism, Vol. 3, Munro, H. N., ed., New York, Academic Press, 1969, p. 189.
41. Rosso, P. Unpublished data.
42. Quirin-Stricker, C., and Mandel, P. Etude du renouvellement en RNA des polysomes, du RNA de transfert et du RNA "messager" dans le foie de rat soumis a un jeune proteique, Bull. Soc. Chim. Biol. 50:13, 1968.
43. Brasel, J. A., Coffey, D. S., and Williams-Ashman, H. G. Androgen induced changes in DNA polymerase activity of coagulating glands of castrated rats, Med. Exp. 18:321, 1969.
44. Brasel, J. A. Age dependent differences in DNA polymerase activity following uninephrectomy in rats, Growth 36:45, 1972.
45. Karp, R., Brasel, J. A., and Winick, M. Compensatory kidney growth after uninephrectomy in adult and infant rats, Amer. J. Dis. Child. 121:186, 1971.
46. Brasel, J. A., Ehrenkranz, R. A., and Winick, M. DNA polymerase activity in rat brain during ontogeny, Develop. Biol. 23:424, 1970.
47. Brasel, J. A., Joh, B. S., and Ehrenkranz, R. A. Patterns of DNA polymerase activity in normal rat forebrain and cerebellum in the suckling period, Growth 37:301, 1973.
48. Jasper, H. G., and Brasel, J. A. Rat liver DNA synthesis in the "catch-up" growth of nutritional rehabilitation, J. Nutr. 104:405, 1974.
49. Metcoff, J. Biochemical markers of intrauterine malnutrition, in Current Concepts in Nutrition, Vol. 2, Nutrition and Fetal Development, Winick, M., ed., New York, John Wiley & Sons, 1974, p. 27.
50. Kraft, N., and Shortman, K. A suggested control function for the animal tissue ribonuclease—ribonuclease inhibitor system, based on studies of

isolated cells and phytohaemagglutinin-transformed lymphocytes, Biochim. Biophys. Acta 217:164, 1970.
51. Rosso, P., and Winick, M. Unpublished observations.
52. Rosso, P., Nelson, M., and Winick, M. Changes in cellular RNA content and alkaline ribonuclease activity in rat liver during development, Growth 37:143, 1973.
53. Rosso, P., and Raguso, L. RNase activity: Rate of RNA degradation and cellular RNA content, Fed. Proc. 31:697, 1972.
54. Rosso, P., and Winick, M. Effects of early undernutrition and subsequent refeeding on alkaline ribonuclease activity on rat cerebrum and liver, J. Nutr., 1975 (in press).
55. Winick, M., and Rosso, P. The effect of severe early malnutrition on cellular growth of human brain, Pediat. Res. 3:181, 1969.
56. Rosso, P., Hormazabal, J., and Winick, M. Changes in brain weight, cholesterol, phospholipid and DNA content in marasmic children, Am. J. Cl. Nutr. 23:1275, 1970.
57. Dickerson, J. Personal communication.

Chapter 4   MALNUTRITION AND PRENATAL GROWTH

NORMAL PLACENTAL GROWTH

The placenta is readily available for study and some abnormalities in fetal growth are reflected in placental growth. With this in mind, investigators have examined placental growth during normal rat pregnancies, normal human pregnancies, and under certain abnormal conditions known to affect the growth of both the rat and the human fetus.

By injecting H^3 thymidine into pregnant rats and employing autoradiography, Jollie was able to demonstrate that labeled mitotic figures do not appear in the trophoblastic layer of the rat placenta after the eighteenth day of pregnancy.[1] In our own studies we could demonstrate that although weight, protein, and RNA content rise linearly until the twentieth day of gestation, DNA content fails to increase after the seventeenth day owing to the cessation of DNA synthesis[2] (Fig. 4-1). Table 1 shows that C^{14} thymidine fails to incorporate into placental DNA between the sixteenth and eighteenth day of pregnancy. It can be noted that during this same period thymidine is rapidly incorporated into the organs

Table 4-1
INCORPORATION OF ^{14}C-THYMIDINE INTO DNA

	Placenta	Embryo
16 days	400 (300–480)	130 (90–180)
18 days	18 (16–20)	550 (480–600)
20 days	18 (16–21)	600 (520–630)
Background	18 (16–20)	18 (16–20)

Figures expressed as c.p.m./mg DNA. Each figure represents the average of ten placentas or embryos. Figures in parentheses represent range.

Source: Winick, M., and Nobel, A. Quantitative changes in ribonucleic acids and protein during normal growth of rat placenta, Nature 212:34, 1966.

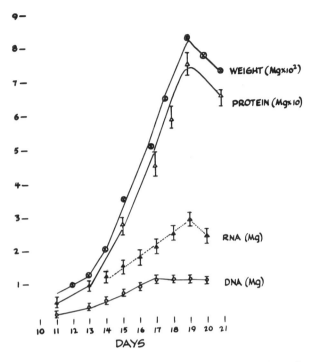

Fig. 4.1. Total weight, protein, DNA, and RNA during development of rat placenta. Each point represents the average of at least fifteen separate determinations. The bars on the figure represent the range.

of the fetus. Hence, cell division stops somewhere around the seventeenth day in rat placenta and the rest of placental growth is due to an increase in protoplasmic elements rather than an increase in cell number. Thus, three phases of cellular growth may be described in rat placenta, just as in other organs of the rat. From 10 days until about 16 days after conception, DNA synthesis and net protein synthesis are proportional, cell number increases, but cell size is unchanged. This is the period of pure hyperplasia. From 16 to 18 days, because of a slowing in the rate of DNA synthesis while protein synthesis continues at the same rate, hyperplasia and hypertrophy are occurring together. Finally, around 18 days, cell division stops altogether. Weight and protein content still continue their linear rise. The weight/DNA or protein/DNA ratios rapidly increase. Hypertrophy is now occurring alone (Fig. 4-2).

Maturational changes occur in the placenta throughout gestation, so

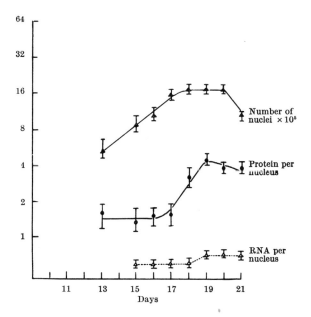

Fig. 4.2. Total organ DNA expressed as number of nuclei and protein/DNA and RNA/DNA ratios expressed as protein or RNA per nucleus in mμg during normal growth of rat placenta

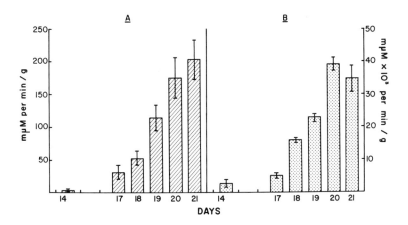

Fig. 4.3. Normal placental transport.

A. Amount of AIB (millimicromoles) transferred across the rat placenta per gram of placental tissue and per minute at different gestational ages. Fetuses were removed 10 minutes after injection of AIB into the mother.

B. Amount of label (expressed as millimicromoles of glucose) transferred across the rat placenta per gram of placental tissue and per minute at different gestational ages. Fetuses were removed 10 minutes after injection of D-glucose-1-(3H) into the mother.

that growth by cell division is not necessary for certain maturational changes to take place. During the final period of hypertrophy certain electron-microscopic changes take place in the rat placenta. There is a reduction of the "placental barrier" with the appearance of endothelial and trophoblastic fenestrations. Increased micropinocytotic activity, irregularities at the inner plasma membrane, and the appearance of large vacuoles can all be seen in the so-called element III. There is also approximation of inner and outer membranes at points of constriction and formation of pedicle-like foot processes.[1]

Concomitant with these morphologic changes, profound functional changes also take place. There is a change in the selectivity of transportable materials and an increase in the transport rate of certain materials. Glycogen, which has previously been deposited in copious amounts, rapidly becomes depleted. There is a marked increase in placental transport in the rat at day 17 of gestation. This has been shown for glucose and alpha amino isobutyric acid transport (Fig. 4-3).

Although the exact timing of events is not as clear as with the rat, available data indicate that the human placenta grows in a qualitatively similar manner. Placenta is the only human tissue in which cellular growth has been studied throughout its entire life span. Therefore, it is not known whether the sequence to be described is characteristic of other human tissues. Studies cited in Chapter 2 indicate, however, that human brain tissue grows in the same way. Data from our laboratory have shown a linear relationship between placental and fetal weight in agreement with the findings of other investigators. We have not been able to study enough fetuses over 3500 grams to exclude the possibility of a terminal falling off in the rate of placental growth as suggested by Gruenwald and Minn.[3] But at least until the fetus reaches 3500 grams, fetal weight gain is accompanied by a linear increase in the weight of the placenta (Fig. 4-4). At the same time it has been shown that total protein and RNA content increases linearly to term. By contrast DNA ceases to increase after the placenta reaches about 300 grams, which corresponds to a fetal weight of about 2400 grams or a gestational age of 34 to 36 weeks[4] (Fig. 4-5). As in the rat, cell division in the human placenta thus ceases before term. Studies by Beaconsfield and her colleagues suggest that this cessation of DNA synthesis is accompanied by a shift in the pathway of glucose metabolism away from the hexosemonophosphate shunt and hence away from nucleic acid synthesis.[5] These changes are reminiscent of the changes in brain tissue described in Chapter 2. Again,

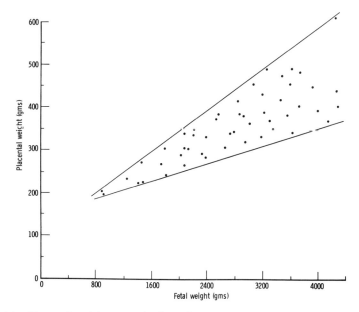

Fig. 4.4.   Placental weight versus fetal weight

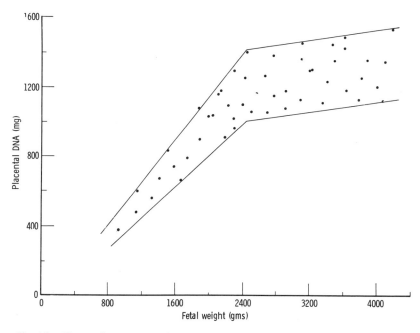

Fig. 4.5.   Placental DNA versus fetal weight

the amount of glucose metabolized through the shunt decreased as the period of proliferative cell growth reached an end.

Although the cellular events are very similar during the growth of human and rat placenta, there is at least one quantitative difference: the RNA/DNA ratio is twice as high in the rat. The reason for this difference is unknown, but it may be due to increased connective tissue within the human placenta.[4] Fibroblasts contain relatively little RNA. Possibly the trophoblasts contain equal quantities of RNA in both species.

Maturation in human placenta also occurs throughout all three growth periods.[6] Again, cell division is not essential to differentiation, either morphologically or functionally. While growth in the two species proceeds for the most part in a similar fashion, differentiation may be quite different at least in certain biochemical aspects. Although both the rat and human placenta lose glycogen as term approaches, there are differences in carbohydrate metabolism, at least *in vitro*. For example, Ginsberg and co-workers have demonstrated that lactic acid production *in vitro* is much greater in rat than in human placenta. Furthermore, adrenaline does not increase lactate production in rat placenta as it does in human placenta.[7] Similarly, glucose uptake is greater in rat placenta and is not enhanced by either anaerobiosis or the addition of adrenaline. Placental glycogen breakdown during incubation is much greater in rat than in human placenta and is not influenced in rat placenta by adding adrenaline.

Since normal cellular growth in the placenta proceeds through an orderly sequence of changes as gestation progresses, the time at which a stimulus is exerted may be as important as the nature of the stimulus itself. A stimulus that interfered with cell division at an early stage might have little or no effect later. Conversely, the nature of the cellular effects produced might give us a clue to the time an unknown stimulus was most active. Experimentally, the DNA, RNA, and protein content of the placenta can be examined under conditions known to affect both fetal and placental growth.

MALNUTRITION AND CELLULAR GROWTH
OF PLACENTA AND FETUS

During intrauterine life all organs of the fetus are in the hyperplastic phase of growth. At no other time should the organism be more susceptible to nutritional stresses, and yet only recently has any information about fetal malnutrition been forthcoming. This is true probably for two reasons, one technical and the other philosophical. The first was the relative inaccessibility of the fetus for experimental manipulation. The second has been the generally accepted view of the fetus as a perfect parasite, extracting what it needs from its mother. Recently, as researchers have begun to explore intrauterine conditions, this view has been challenged. Fetal malnutrition may result from reduced maternal circulation, inadequate nutrients within the maternal circulation, or faulty placental transport of specific nutrients. The first two situations are now being extensively investigated in laboratory animals.

Reduction of blood supply

The supply of blood to a single fetus in an animal delivering a litter of fetuses may be reduced spontaneously. It is not uncommon to see a "runt" in a litter of dogs or cats, and it is common knowledge that these animals will survive only with special care and that they will never reach the same final size as their litter mates even if this special care is given. Occasionally the same situation occurs in a litter of pigs, and Widdowson has studied the cellular changes that take place in the organs of these runt pigs. Her findings indicate that cell division is curtailed and cell size reduced in the heart, kidney, brain, and skeletal muscle, the only organs she has studied so far.[8]

In the rat, blood supply can be artificially reduced by clamping the uterine artery supplying one uterine horn (Fig. 4-6). Using this technique, Wigglesworth has compared the growth of fetuses in the ligated horn to that of the fetuses in the unligated horn.[9] Growth rate was reduced in proportion to the distance of the fetus from the ligated artery. Those closest to the ligation generally died. As one progressed farther away from the ligated uterine artery and closer to the intact ovarian artery, the growth rate increased. More recently, the cellular growth of the placenta and various fetal organs has been studied in the surviving animals within the ligated horn. Ligation on the thirteenth day of gestation will affect the rate of cell division in the placenta and the fetal organs. Ligation on the seventeenth day will again curtail cell division in the fetal organs, but in the placenta cell size will be reduced while cell number remains normal.[10] The placenta thus responds in a manner that might

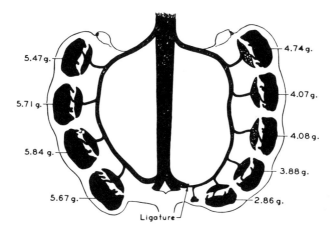

Fig. 4.6. Method of producing vascular insufficiency in pregnant rats. Schematic diagram of the experimental model. The fetal weights were taken from one experiment.

have been predicted from other studies of early postnatal malnutrition; ligation during the period of hyperplasia results in a reduced cell number, whereas ligation during hypertrophy results in reduced cell size. By determining the final effect on placental growth at delivery, it may therefore be possible to pinpoint the time at which malnutrition occurred. As we shall see, this may be useful in research on malnutrition in humans, where placenta is the only tissue readily available for study.

Our own studies have defined another abnormality in placentas from the ligated horns. After an initial elevation of total organ RNA content and hence an elevation of the RNA/DNA ratio or RNA per cell, there was a drop in the total RNA content and a reduced RNA/DNA ratio.[10] Such initial elevations have been described in several tissues under a variety of circumstances: clamping the aorta results in an increased RNA/DNA ratio in the left ventricle;[11] repeated nerve stimulation results in an initial elevation of the RNA/DNA ratio in the innervated muscle;[12] injection of estrogen results in an initial increase in the RNA/DNA ratio in the uterus; and removal of one kidney initially increases the RNA/DNA ratio in the contralateral kidney.[13] The exact significance of this change is unknown but it has been described under conditions requiring increased protein synthesis. The increase in the placental RNA/DNA ratio may therefore represent an abortive attempt by placental cells to increase their rate of protein synthesis in response to the stress of vascular insufficiency. Careful examination of the fetus reveals that the cellular growth of certain organs is disproportionately affected by interference with the placental blood supply. In the liver there is approximately a 50% reduction in DNA content. In the brain, however, there is little or no effect on the number of cells[10] (Table 4-2). Some clinicians have suggested that this disproportionate effect on liver and brain size accounts for the type of intrauterine growth retardation that results in small-for-dates infants who have a small, depleted liver and a normal-size brain. They further postulate that it is this type of fetus which is most prone to neonatal hypoglycemia since the liver is unable to supply to the brain the nutrients which it requires. Whether this interpretation is correct remains to be seen. Similar findings have recently been reported in monkeys.[14] Ablation of a portion of the placenta to produce "placental insufficiency" sharply retarded the fetal growth rate. Again, the liver and skeletal muscle were markedly affected, showing a reduced number of cells and reduced RNA and protein content per cell. The brain was hardly affected at all. Only slight changes in the RNA content of the cerebellum could be demonstrated. The "undernutrition" produced by vascular insufficiency thus results in asymmetrical type of growth failure in which the brain is relatively spared. It has been demonstrated recently that this is probably due to reflex vasodilation in the arteries supplying the fetal brain, which sets up a preferential blood supply for that organ and further depletes other organs.[15]

Table 4-2
EFFECT ON FETAL TISSUES OF UTERINE ARTERY
LIGATION ON THE SEVENTEENTH DAY OF GESTATION

Tissue	Weight	% Normal Control Protein	RNA	DNA
Whole Animal	67	71	63	71
Brain	91	95	104	99
Heart	84	84	79	91
Lung	62	65	55	59
Liver	62	70	75	55
Kidney	64	61	82	75

Source: Winick, M., Brasel, J. A., and Rosso, P. Nutrition and cell growth, in Current Concepts in Nutrition, Vol. 1, Nutrition and Development, Winick, M., ed., New York, John Wiley & Sons, 1972.

MATERNAL PROTEIN RESTRICTION

It is also possible to retard placental and fetal growth by restricting protein in the maternal diet of rats. The cellular changes produced by severe prenatal food restriction are reflected in the placenta earlier than in the fetus, but retardation of cell division in all fetal organs can be clearly demonstrated.[10] In the placenta, cell number (DNA content) was reduced by 13 days after conception, cell size (protein/DNA ratio) remained normal, and the RNA/DNA ratio again shows an abortive increase (Table 4-3). The retardation in fetal growth first became apparent at 15 days. After that there was a progressive decrease in cell number in all organs studied. The reduction in brain cell number is proportional to the reduction in the number of cells in the other organs. By term, brain cell number was only 85% of normal (Table 4-4). These findings agree with those of Zamenhof, who found a similar reduction in total brain cell number in term fetuses whose mothers were exposed to a slightly different type of nutritional deprivation.[16] This type of fetal growth retardation differs from that which is produced by vascular insufficiency as it is a proportional reduction in the size of all organs. A small liver supplies a small brain, and it is postulated that in this type of intrauterine growth failure the fetus is much less susceptible to the effects of neonatal hypoglycemia. The reduction in brain cell number in these fetuses, however, is different from that which is seen with postnatal malnutrition. By using

Table 4-3
EFFECT OF MATERNAL MALNUTRITION ON PLACENTA*

	Control	Experimental
Weight	.405	.320
Protein	28.0	21.7
RNA	1.00	1.80
DNA	1.06	0.82
RNA/DNA	0.99	2.1
Prot/DNA	27.0	28.2

* Data expressed in Mg. per whole placenta.

Source: Winick, M., Brasel, J. A., and Rosso, P. Nutrition and cell growth, in Current Concepts in Nutrition, Vol. 1, Nutrition and Development, Winick, M., ed., New York, John Wiley & Sons, 1972.

Table 4-4

EFFECT OF MATERNAL MALNUTRITION ON FETAL TISSUES

Tissue	Weight	% Normal Control Protein	RNA	DNA
Whole Animal	87	81	83	81
Brain	91	85	82	84
Heart	84	84	79	81
Lung	82	85	85	89
Liver	82	80	85	85
Kidney	84	81	82	85

Source: Winick, M., Brasel, J. A., and Rosso, P. Nutrition and cell growth, in Current Concepts in Nutrition, Vol. 1, Nutrition and Development, Winick, M., ed., New York, John Wiley & Sons, 1972.

autoradiography after injecting the mother with tritiated thymidine, one can assess cell division in various discrete brain regions.[10] Differential regional sensitivity to maternal protein restriction can be demonstrated in this way by the sixteenth day of gestation in the brains of fetuses of protein-restricted mothers. The cerebral white and gray matter are both mildly affected. The area adjacent to the third ventricle and the subiculum is moderately affected, while the cerebellum and the area directly adjacent to the lateral ventricle are markedly affected (Fig. 4-7). These findings again demonstrate that the magnitude of the effect of malnutrition depends largely on the rate of cell division. Moreover, they demonstrate that the maternal placental barrier in the rat is not effective in protecting the fetal brain from discrete cellular effects caused by maternal food restriction.

The subsequent course of the animals born of protein-restricted mothers can be examined. Chow reported that even if these animals are raised normally by foster mothers their ability to utilize nitrogen is permanently impaired.[17] In our own laboratory we have found that if such animals are nursed by normal foster mothers in normal-size litters, they will still have a deficit in total brain cell number at weaning.[10] These same newborn pups of protein-restricted mothers may be subjected to postnatal nutritional manipulation. If they are raised in litters of 3 by normal foster mothers until weaning, the deficit in their total number of brain cells may be almost entirely reversed.[18] Although the number of cells approaches normal, the deficit at birth might very well be made up by later increases in cell number in areas other than those most affected *in utero*.

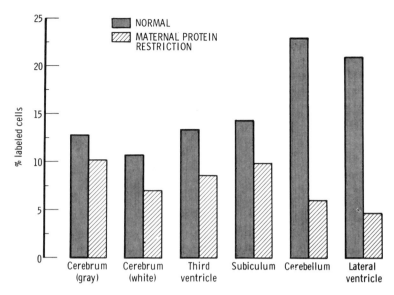

Fig. 4.7. DNA content of various regions in developing rat brain

Although it may appear that optimally nourishing pups after exposing them to prenatal undernutrition will reverse the cellular effects, this may not actually be so in specific brain areas.

Perhaps the experimental situation that offers the closest analogue to the realities of human malnutrition is the exposure of pups malnourished *in utero* to subsequent postnatal deprivation. The effects of such exposure or deprivation on brain cell morphology, as described for the dog in the preceding section, are extreme: a marked degeneration of certain neuronal elements and an increase in gliosis, especially in the spinal cord and the medullary areas of the puppies. These changes are not reversed when the puppies are rehabilitated. If rats are raised in litters of 18 after having been malnourished *in utero,* they will suffer a 60% reduction in total brain cell number by the time of weaning.[19] This is much more pronounced than the effect of either prenatal or postnatal under-nutrition alone. Rats subjected to prenatal malnutrition alone showed a 15% reduction in total brain cell number at birth. Rats subjected to postnatal malnutrition alone showed a reduction of 15 to 20% of their brain cells by weaning (Fig. 4-8). These data demonstrate that malnutrition applied constantly throughout the entire period of brain cell proliferation will result in a profound reduction in brain cell number, greater

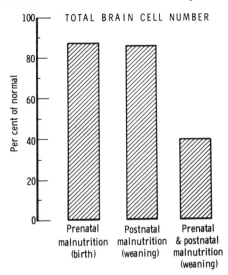

TOTAL BRAIN CELL NUMBER

Fig. 4.8. Comparison of food restriction after birth, protein restriction during gestation, and "combined" prenatal and postnatal restriction

than the sum of effects produced during various parts of the proliferative phase. It appears that the duration of malnutrition as well as the severity during this early critical period is extremely important in determining the ultimate cellular make-up of the brain.

Recent experiments by Widdowson demonstrate that caloric restriction in the guinea pig during gestation markedly reduces the birth weight of the offspring and curtails the rate of cell division in the brain.[8] In the skeletal muscle not only is there a reduction in cell number, but the actual number of muscle fibers is reduced and each muscle fiber has an increased number of nuclei. When fed normally after birth, these animals fail to recover normal height and weight. In a variety of animal species, then, severe protein restriction during gestation produces manifestations similar to those of malnutrition during the early postnatal period. In addition, malnutrition prolonged through the periods of gestation and lactation has much more severe consequences on the cellular growth. Recent findings by Barnes and his colleagues have shown that these "doubly deprived" animals not only are permanently impaired in their food efficiency but also have abnormalities in oxygen consumption which persist even after long-term rehabilitation.[20]

SPECIFIC NUTRIENT DEFICIENCIES

In the previous section we have been discussing the effects of a reduction in either total calories or total protein on the nutrition and subsequent growth of the fetus. Deficiencies in specific nutrients may also affect fetal development.

Reduced levels of vitamin A have long been known to be teratogenic in the rat. Experiments in our laboratory have demonstrated that marginal vitamin A deficiency in the mother will retard growth in the fetus. By 16 days of gestation the earliest effects of this growth failure can be detected in the placenta, where the number of cells is reduced.[21]

Another vitamin whose deficiency is known to affect the developing brain in both humans and experimental animals is vitamin B_6. Newborn infants accidentally subjected to a deficiency of this vitamin had convulsive seizures which were cured by administration of the vitamin.[22] These infants also had grossly abnormal electroencephalograms. The precise biochemical alterations in the brain are not known, but since B_6 is a coenzyme in many essential reactions it is not surprising that profound metabolic disturbances result from its deficiency. In newborn rats, vitamin B_6 deficiency reduces the rate of DNA synthesis and the number of cells in the brain.[23]

Another vitamin deficiency recently implicated in abnormal brain development is that of folic acid. Evidence suggests that folic acid deficiency induced in the mother by certain drugs, such as dilantin, will result in an increased number of congenital malformations.[24] This deficiency is also accompanied by abnormal electroencephalograms in the offspring.

There has been increasing concern over the role of heavy metals during pregnancy. Hurley has shown that zinc, manganese, and perhaps magnesium deficiency during pregnancy may all have adverse effects on the fetus.[25] Zinc deficiency can be induced extremely rapidly in the rat by withholding zinc from the maternal diet. When this is done during the entire period of pregnancy, almost all fetuses are malformed and the malformations involve almost every organ system. Even if the deficiency is restricted to the time between the sixth and fourteenth day of gestation, half the fetuses are malformed and stunted in growth. The growth retardation is accompanied by a decreased rate of cell division as measured by decrease in thymidine uptake. These findings take on more significance in view of reported zinc deficiencies in human populations. In contrast to zinc deficiency, manganese deficiency does not result in obvious malformations. The most striking effect of manganese deficiency in the maternal diet during pregnancy is an irreversible congenital ataxia in the offspring. This ataxia is secondary to faulty otolith development which may come about because of faulty mucopolysaccharide synthesis. Preliminary data suggest that magnesium deficiency also may result in serious malformations of the fetus.

Excesses of certain heavy metals both prenatally and immediately postnatally lead to impairment of brain growth. When 25 ppm of lead is placed in the drinking water of pregnant rats from conception until their pups are weaned, cell division in the developing brain is curtailed so that the brains of such pups show a 20% reduction in DNA content. Similar findings occur when 1 ppm of methyl mercury is put in the drinking water. In both of these situations no demonstrable effect on the adult brain is present. Thus again we can see the extreme sensitivity of the *developing* brain to an environmental stimulus—in this case a heavy metal.

MALNUTRITION AND CELLULAR GROWTH OF THE HUMAN PLACENTA

Like the organs of the rat, the human placenta goes through three phases of growth. Cell division ceases at about 34 to 36 weeks of gestation while weight and protein increase nearly until term.[4] Placentas from infants that had suffered intrauterine growth failure (probably due to vascular insufficiency) showed fewer cells and an increased RNA/DNA ratio when compared to control placentas.[26] Fifty per cent of placentas from an indigent population in Chile showed similar effects. Placentas from a malnourished population in Guatemala had fewer cells than normal placentas. In a single case of anorexia nervosa in which a severely emaciated mother carried to term and gave birth to a 2000 gm infant, the placenta contained less than 50% of the expected number of cells[10] (Fig. 4-9). Thus both vascular insufficiency and maternal malnutrition will curtail cell division in human placenta. The cellular make-up of the placenta in both of these situations strongly suggests that both stimuli

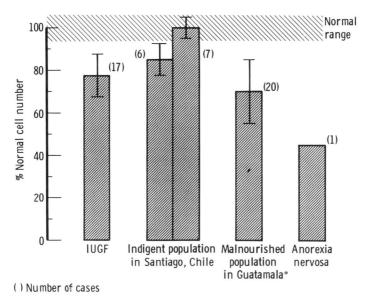

Fig. 4.9. Comparison of placental DNA content in various types of maternal deprivation

have been active for some time prior to the thirty-fourth to thirty-sixth week of gestation.

Fetal nutrition depends on the size and functional capacity of the trophoblast and on the villous surface area through which the exchange of nutrients takes place. Accordingly, rather than simply expressing data in terms of total RNA and DNA, some authors have compared various morphological characteristics of placentas from well-nourished (Boston) and poorly nourished (Guatemala City) women.[27] Both fetal and placental weight were considerably reduced in the Guatemalan population. Morphometric analysis of the well-nourished placentas indicated that only 12% of the placental weight consisted of trophoblast, which is thought to be the most important part of the placenta, in terms of metabolic function. The villous mass, trophoblastic mass, and villous surface areas of the peripheral villi were significantly lower in the Guatemalan group. The trophoblastic mass was 58 grams in the well-nourished placentas and only 43 grams in the poorly nourished placentas. The decrease in mass seemed to depend on a reduction in the number of peripheral villi rather than a reduction in the size of the individual villus. Furthermore, the stem villi do not take part in this decrease, and both their trophoblastic mass (which represents about 1/20 of the total trophoblastic mass) and their fibroblastic mass (which represents about 1/5 of the total fibroblastic mass) are statistically indistinguishable in the two groups. This suggests that the growth and maturation of the peripheral villi are more sensitive to maternal malnutrition than the growth and maturation of the stem villi. In fact, the trophoblastic mass of the stem villi had a tendency to be greater in the placentas of the poorly nourished mothers than in those of the well-nourished mothers. Along with the reduced trophoblastic mass in the poorly nourished placentas, there was a concomitant reduction in total surface areas of the peripheral villi and of their capillaries. Such reductions limit the surface over which physiologic exchange can take place. There were no similar reductions in the case of the stem villi, but rather a significant increase in the capillary bed of the stem villi, possibly a compensatory factor in nutrient exchange. The higher incidence and extent of both old and new infarcts among the malnourished placentas and the significantly higher proportion of intervillous space taken up by fibrin in these placentas suggest disturbances in placental circulation and the coagulation of fibrinolytic systems during pregnancy in the malnourished mothers. In addition, certain pathological features were present in greater number in the placentas of malnourished mothers. These included circumvallation and succenturiate lobes within the placenta. Thus malnutrition results in a reduction in functional tissue and in surface area for exchange both at the villous surfaces and at the surfaces of the capillaries of peripheral villi. Without first evaluating the functional capacity of the placentas, however, no causal relationship between these placental deficits and fetal development can be established. A biochemical analysis of these placentas was also performed, but findings did not reflect the 25% reduction in total mass of active placental tissue (combined trophoblastic and fibroblastic masses of the villi) in the malnourished placentas. The insensitivity of these particular parameters in differentiating between the two series of placentas is, of course, due to the necessity of using samples containing the mixed tissues of the placenta, some of which are not responsive to the changes seen in the peripheral villi of the malnourished placentas. Although the differences in this series were not statistically significant, there was a tendency toward a reduced DNA content in the placentas of the malnourished group. The authors concluded that since placental DNA content does not increase after 36 weeks of gestation, the differences noted were due to either failure of cell division before that time or actual cell death. All of the other chemical constituents measured when expressed per whole placenta were lower in the Guatemalan than in the Boston population. Average placental RNA was reduced and average placental protein content was also reduced. In addition, heat-stable alkaline phosphatase activity was less in the malnourished placentas.

The effects of prenatal stimuli on the cellular growth of the fetus are more difficult to assess. Indirect evidence suggests that cell division in the human fetus may be inhibited by maternal undernutrition, so that fetal growth is retarded and birth weight reduced. If one examines the available information on infants who died after exposure to severe postnatal malnutrition, three patterns emerge. Breast-fed infants malnourished during the second year have a reduced protein/DNA ratio but a normal brain DNA content. Full-term infants who died of severe food deprivation during the first year of life show a 15 to 20% reduction in total brain cell number. Infants weighing 2000 gm or less at birth who died of severe undernutrition during the first year of life show a 60% reduction in total brain cell number[19] (Fig. 4-10). It is possible that the children in this last category were deprived *in utero* and represent a clinical counterpart of the "doubly deprived" animal. It is also possible that these were true premature infants and that the premature is much more susceptible to postnatal malnutrition than the full-term infant. At the present time it is impossible to differentiate between these two possibilities because of the lack of adequate data on gestational age. Regardless of which of these two possibilities turns out to be correct, however, it is important that in certain countries in the developing world and among certain populations in our own country 20% of the infants born may fall into this low birth weight category.

NEWER APPROACHES TO THE STUDY
OF FETAL MALNUTRITION

In the previous chapter, a number of biochemical changes in brain and liver were described in young animals subjected to malnutrition. These changes reflected metabolic alterations in the tissues and have helped provide some insight into certain of the mechanisms involved in produc-

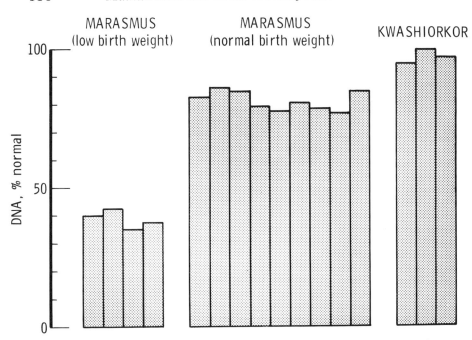

Fig. 4.10. Comparison of brain cell number in marasmus, marasmus plus low birth weight, and kwashiorkor

ing the cellular effects of early malnutrition. In addition, however, it has recently been shown that some of these changes, because of their magnitude, can be measured in the placenta and fetus of animals subjected to experimental prenatal malnutrition and in the human placenta in malnourished populations.

As we have seen, at least two types of intrauterine malnutrition exist. One type produces obvious changes in cellular growth of the fetal brain, whereas the other produces little if any change in fetal brain when measurements of weight, protein, RNA, and DNA content are made. (As we shall see, however, more subtle changes can be measured by newer biochemical parameters.) These two types of fetal malnutrition do not, as far as we can tell at present, depend on the species employed but rather on the method by which the malnutrition is induced. For example "placental insufficiency" will result in retarded fetal growth. This condition has been produced by ligating the uterine artery in rats and more recently by ablating a portion of the placenta in monkeys.[9, 14] In the rat such a ligation produces a reduction in weight, protein, RNA, and DNA content in placenta and most fetal tissues. Brain, however, is unaffected. The same is apparently the case in the monkey following ablation of a portion of the placenta. Using such a model, Cheek and his collaborators have demonstrated that although profound fetal growth failure will occur, brain weight, protein, and DNA content are unaffected and RNA content is reduced only about 5% in cerebellum.[14] This relatively small reduction may become more significant when taken together with more recent data examining other tissue parameters. Thus both in the rat and in the monkey this type of placental insufficiency results in a markedly disproportionate type of growth failure in which brain is relatively spared and organs such as liver markedly affected.

If we now re-examine this model using some of the newer markers of tissue nutritional status, certain changes not previously seen become obvious.[28] Within 24 hours after ligation a marked elevation of placental RNase activity can be demonstrated. Enzyme activity increases in inverse proportion to the distance from the ligation. There is a marked elevation in the proximal placenta, a milder elevation in intermediately located placentas and minimal changes in those located distally (Fig. 4-11). If we limit our observations to the proximal placenta, alkaline RNase activity is elevated within 24 hours and remains elevated for at least 96 hours (Fig. 4-12). This increase in activity precedes any changes in placental weight, protein, DNA, or RNA content. In the fetal organs, there is a marked increase in liver RNase within 24 hours, with brain unaffected. By 48 hours, however, both brain and liver RNase are distinctly elevated (Fig. 4-13). Thus, by examining activity of alkaline RNase, changes in brain can be demonstrated after 48 hours of ligation in the absence of any reduction in weight, protein, DNA, or RNA content. These data become even more interesting when coupled with the observations of Cheek and associates in the monkey.[14] Although these investigators did not measure alkaline RNase activity, their demonstration of a slight reduction in cerebellar RNA content may be more meaningful in this context. At present, then, the available data suggest that this type of placental insufficiency will produce certain changes in RNA metabolism of fetal brain without permanently affecting cellular growth as measured by brain weight, protein, or nucleic acid content. What the significance, if any, of this increased enzyme activity is remains to be determined.

In contrast to the placental insufficiency model, maternal protein restriction in rats, pigs, and guinea pigs produces a symmetrical reduction

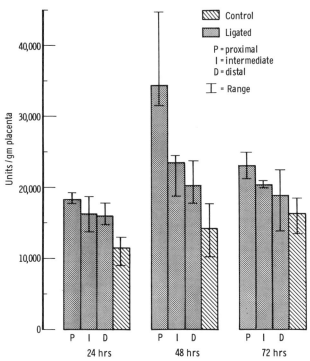

Fig. 4.11. Changes in RNase activity in rat placenta 24, 48, and 72 hours after uterine artery ligation. Enzyme activity in general increases inversely with the distance from the ligation.

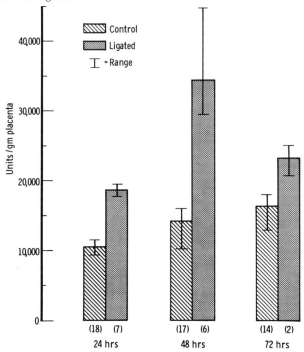

Fig. 4.12. RNase activity in proximal placentas following ligation of the uterine artery

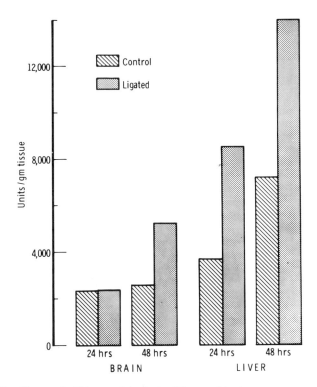

Fig. 4.13.   Changes in RNase activity in fetal liver and brain

in weight, protein, RNA, and DNA content of all organs including brain. Thus in this type of fetal malnutrition the brain is not spared. If we now turn to measurement of our more recently described markers of tissue nutritional status, we can demonstrate first that activity of DNA polymerase parallels the rate of cell division during normal placental growth and that this type of maternal malnutrition will result in reduced activity of this enzyme in placenta by 12 days of gestation (Fig. 4-14). Moreover alkaline RNase activity is markedly elevated in such placentas (Fig. 4-15). Thus activity of both DNA polymerase and alkaline RNase has proved a sensitive index of nutritional status, at least in placenta, in rats exposed to maternal protein restriction.

How can these changes provide us with clinically useful tools for the assessment of nutritional status? DNA polymerase activity has recently been measured in human leukocytes and has been shown to increase markedly in situations of abnormally rapid cell division such as leuke-

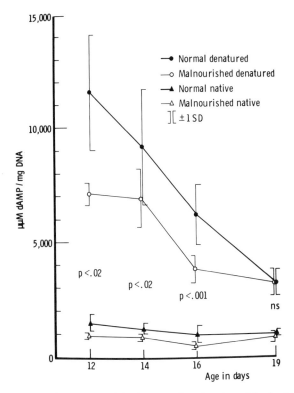

Fig. 4.14.   DNA polymerase activity in normal and malnourished rat placenta

mia.[19] Moreover this increased activity precedes by several days any increase in leukocyte cell number and has been used to predict recurrence of disease after drug-induced remission. The possibility exists that enzyme activity may be reduced in leukocytes of malnourished children and that activity might increase with therapy. In addition, since it has been shown that DNA polymerase activity parallels the rate of cell division in tissues other than brain, activity in a muscle biopsy could give us a quantitative measure of the rate of cell division in muscle of malnourished children. Finally, since activity of this enzyme is reduced in placenta in experimental malnutrition, perhaps it will also be reduced in placentas of malnourished women. Already assay requirements have been worked out and activity measured in normal human placenta.[30]

As previously mentioned, Metcoff and colleagues are actively examining leukocytes and placenta for RNA polymerase activity in populations

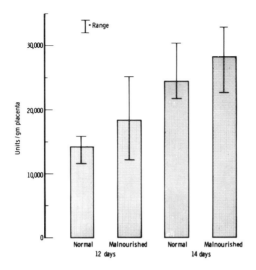

Fig. 4.15. Alkaline RNase activity in malnourished rat placenta

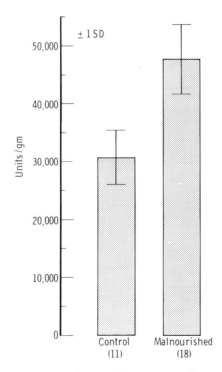

Fig. 4.16. Total RNase activity in human placentas—Ecuador

of malnourished women.[31] It is hoped that their investigations will also sharpen our tools for assessing nutritional status.

We have recently focused our attention on alkaline RNase as a clinically useful marker of nutritional status. Examination of placentas of a group of malnourished mothers in Quito, Ecuador, revealed an elevated RNase activity when compared to placentas from normally nourished women in the same city[32] (Fig. 4-16). This enzyme is not only present in all tissues but is found in normal plasma and normal urine and we have measured it in normal amniotic fluid. Obviously changes in the activity of this enzyme in any of these fluids would provide a practical approach to the monitoring of either postnatal or prenatal nutritional status. Plasma RNase exists almost entirely in the free form, and during development the activity of this enzyme per milliliter of plasma decreases[33] (Fig. 4-17). Enzyme activity was significantly increased in plasma from 14 malnourished children when compared to age-matched controls. Moreover, plasma activity returned to normal after only 2 weeks of therapy in all cases[33] (Fig. 4-18). Sometimes this return to normal preceded any noticeable weight gain in these children.

These results were obtained in severely malnourished children. In such children not only is the serum RNase elevated but the urine RNase is also increased since normal kidney reabsorption of this enzyme is impaired. Children with milder degrees of malnutrition (Grade 1 or 2) also show elevated serum RNase activity but the urine RNase is normal since reabsorption is not impaired. All degrees of malnutrition in children thus produce elevated serum RNase activity. The urinary plasma ratio (U/P) is high in severe (Grade 3) malnutrition and within the normal range in Grades 1 and 2 malnutrition, however. It is therefore possible that by using both serum and urinary RNase measurements we will be able to determine the extent and severity of malnutrition in a susceptible population[33] (Fig. 4-19). In addition, measurements of this enzyme activity in serum should provide a means for monitoring the effectiveness of rehabilitative therapy.

Urea excretion has been used as a rough measure of the rate of protein synthesis and degradation. Studies in Jamaica and in Africa have indicated that urea excretion in severely malnourished children is reduced.[34, 35] Since amniotic fluid is composed largely of fetal urine, we have studied urea concentration in rat amniotic fluid during normal development and after uterine artery ligation. The data indicate an increase in urea concentration during normal development and a marked reduc-

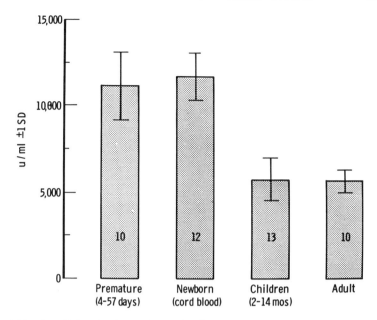

Fig. 4.17.   Free RNase in plasma during development

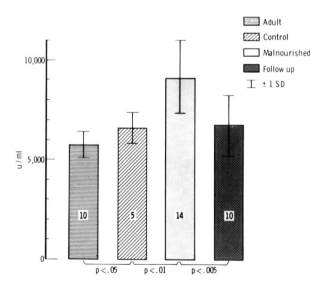

Fig. 4.18.   Plasma RNase—malnutrition and recovery

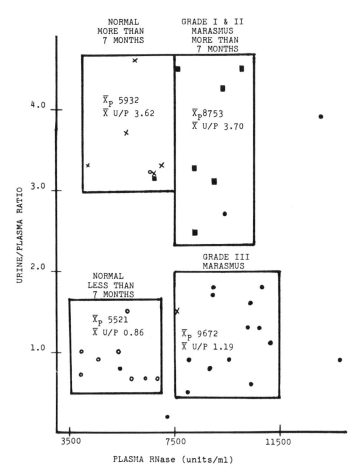

Fig. 4.19. Plasma and urine RNase values in malnourished children. Plasma levels are equal in normal children regardless of age. Children over 7 months have a mean urine/plasma ratio above 3.0, whereas younger infants have a ratio of approximately 1.0. All malnourished children have elevated plasma RNase levels. The less severely ill children have normal urine/plasma ratios, whereas the severely marasmic infants have a low urine/plasma ratio. The means for each group are noted in each of the boxes that have been drawn free hand in order to encompass the majority of points for each group. Open squares represent normal infants 7 to 14 months of age. Closed squares represent infants from 7 to 14 months of age with grades I and II malnutrition; closed circles, infants from 2 to 48 months with grade III malnutrition.

tion following uterine artery clamping in fetuses indicating 25% or greater reduction in body weight.[36]

The task before us remains very large: to diagnose and treat fetal malnutrition *before* the infant is born. We have only begun to search for the diagnostic tools. But the search has already been productive and can be expected to be even more so in the future. Perhaps the use of a battery of these biochemical tests in maternal serum, urine, and amniotic fluid will allow future physicians to identify women who are malnourished and whose fetuses as a consequence are growing poorly. If this occurs the way will be open to specific therapy in specific pregnancies. Until this occurs we must intensify our efforts to see to it that all women are adequately nourished both before and during pregnancy.

REFERENCES

1. Jollie, W. P. Radioautographic observations on variations in desoxyribonucleic acid synthesis in rat placenta with increasing gestational age, Amer. J. Anat. 114:161, 1964.
2. Winick, M., and Noble, A. Quantitative changes in ribonucleic acids and protein during normal growth of rat placenta, Nature 212:34, 1966.
3. Gruenwald, P., and Minn, H. N. Evaluation of body and organ weights in perinatal pathology. II. Weight of body and placenta of surviving and of autopsied infants, Amer. J. Obstet. Gynec. 82:312, 1961.
4. Winick, M., Coscia, A., and Noble, A. Cellular growth in human placenta. I. Normal placental growth, Pediatrics 39:248, 1967.
5. Beaconsfield, P., Ginsburg, J., and Jeacock, M. Glucose metabolism via the pentose phosphate pathway relative to nucleic acid and protein synthesis in the human placenta, Develop. Med. Child. Neurol. 6:469, 1964.
6. Hagerman, D. C., and Villee, C. A. Transport functions of the placenta, Physiol. Rev. 40:313, 1960.
7. Ginsburg, J., and Jeacock, M. Some aspects of placental carbohydrate metabolism in rat, Biochem. Pharmacol. 16:497, 1967.
8. Widdowson, E. M. Reported at Symposium on Fetal Malnutrition sponsored by the National Foundation, March of Dimes, New York City, January 1970.
9. Wigglesworth, J. S. Experimental growth retardation in the foetal rat, J. Pathol. Bacteriol. 88:1, 1964.
10. Winick, M., Brasel, J. A., and Rosso, P. Nutrition and cell growth, in Current Concepts in Nutrition, Vol. 1, Nutrition and Development, Winick, M., ed., New York, John Wiley & Sons, 1972, p. 49.

11. Gluck, L., Talner, N. J., Stern, H., Gardner, T. H., and Kulovich, M. V. Experimental cardiac hypertrophy: Concentrations of RNA in the ventricles, Sci. 144:1244, 1964.

12. Lagan, J. E., Mannell, W. A., and Rossiter, R. J. Chemical studies of peripherae nerve during Wallerian degeneration, J. Biochem. 51:482, 1952.

13. Karp, R., Brasel, J. A., and Winick, M. Compensatory kidney growth after uninephrectomy in adult and infant rats, Amer. J. Dis. Child. 121:186, 1971.

14. Hill, D. E., Wyers, R. E., Holt, A. B., Scott, R. E., and Cheek, D. B. Fetal growth retardation produced by experimental placental insufficiency in Rhesus monkey. II. Chemical composition of the brain, liver, muscle and carcass, Biol. Neonat. 19:68, 1971.

15. Minkowski, A., Roux, J-M., and Tordet-Caridroit, C. Pathophysiologic changes in intrauterine malnutrition, in Current Concepts in Nutrition, Vol. 2, Nutrition and Fetal Development, Winick, M., ed., New York, John Wiley & Sons, 1974, p. 45.

16. Zamenhof, S., Van Martens, F., and Margolis, F. L. DNA (cell number) and protein in neonatal brain: Alteration by maternal dietary protein restriction, Sci. 160:322, 1968.

17. Chow, B. F., and Lees, C. J. Effect of dietary restriction of pregnant rats on body weight gain of the offspring, J. Nutr. 82:10, 1964.

18. Winick, M. Cellular changes during placental and fetal growth, Amer. J. Obstet. Gynec. 109:166, 1971.

19. Winick, M. Nutrition and nerve cell growth, Fed. Proc. 29:1510, 1970.

20. Barnes, R. A. Personal communication.

21. Takahashi, Y. I., and Smith, J. E. Prenatal biochemical changes in vitamin A deficient rats given retinoic acid, Fed. Proc., 32: No. 3, Part 1, 910 Abs., March 1973.

22. Coursin, D. B. Effects of vitamin B_6 on the central nervous activity in chilhood, Amer. J. Cl. Nutr. 4:354, 1956.

23. Bhagavan, H. N., and Coursin, D. B. Effect of pyridoxine deficiency on nucleic acid and protein contents of brain and liver in rats, Intl. J. Vitam. Res. 41:419, 1971.

24. Arakawa, T., Honda, Y., and Narisawa, K. Mechanism of decrease in serum folate levels of rats with diphenylhydantoin administration, Tokohu J. Exp. Med. 111:203, 1973.

25. Hurley, L. Reported at Symposium on Fetal Malnutrition sponsored by the National Foundation, March of Dimes, New York City, January 1970.

26. Winick, M., and Noble, A. Cellular growth in human placenta. II. Diabetes Mellitus, J. Pediat. 71:216, 1967.

27. Laga, E. M., Driscoll, S. G., and Munro, H. N. Comparison of placentas from two socioeconomic groups. I. Morphometry. Pediatrics 50:33, 1972.

28. Velasco, E. G., Brasel, J. A., Sigulem, D. M., Rosso, P., and Winick, M.

Effects of vascular insufficiency on placental ribonuclease activity in the rat, J. Nutr. 103:213, 1973.

29. Gulati, S. C., Axel, R., and Spiegelman, S. Detection of RNA-instructed DNA polymerase and high molecular weight RNA in malignant tissue. Proc. Nat. Acad. Sci., U.S.A. 69:2020, 1972.

30. Velasco, E. G., Brasel, J. A., and Winick, M. Cellular growth of placenta and fetus during prenatal malnutrition, in Western Hemisphere Nutrition Congress III, Miami Beach, 1971, Proc., Mt. Kisco, New York, Futura Publ., 1972, p. 336.

31. Metcoff, J. Fetal malnutrition in biochemical markers of intrauterine malnutrition in Current Concepts in Nutrition, Vol. 2, Nutrition and Fetal Development, Winick, M., ed., New York, John Wiley & Sons, 1974, p. 27.

32. Velasco, E. G., Rosso, P., Brasel, J. A., and Winick, M. Activity of alkaline RNase in placentas of malnourished women, J. Obstet. Gynec. 1975 (in press).

33. Sigulem, D. M., Brasel, J. A., Velasco, E. G., Rosso, P., and Winick, M. Plasma and urine RNase as a measure of nutritional status in children, Amer. J. Clin. Nutr. 26:793, 1973.

34. Alleyne, G. A. O., Flores, H., Picou, D. I. M., and Waterlow, J. C. Metabolic changes in children with protein-calorie malnutrition, in Current Concepts in Nutrition, Vol. 1, Nutrition and Development, Winick, M., ed., New York, John Wiley & Sons, 1972, p. 201.

35. Whitehead, R. G. Biochemical changes in kwashiorkor and nutritional marasmus, in Calorie Deficiencies and Protein Deficiencies, McCance, R. A., and Widdowson, E. M., eds., London, J. and A. Churchill, Ltd., 1968.

Chapter 5 **MALNUTRITION AND
MENTAL DEVELOPMENT**

INTRODUCTION

Over the past 15 years, several studies involving different scientific disciplines have pointed to an association between malnutrition during a critical period of development and permanent changes in brain function. This association has been described in complex human situations that do not permit isolation of any single causal factor. As we have seen, malnutrition usually occurs in a milieu where low socio-economic status, limited education, poor sanitary conditions, and recurrent infections are common. In an attempt to isolate the nutrition factor and to explore the interrelations between malnutrition and other aspects of this environment, a number of epidemiological surveys of human populations have been made, and animal models have been sought. The human studies have the obvious advantage of immediate relevance. In addition psychological testing of children is highly developed and well standardized and there is a voluminous literature existing on the interpretation of many psychological tests. But human studies suffer from the same limitations in interpretation as do animal studies when the testing is done on very young infants. The younger the child, the more difficult it is to use the results of any test as an index of future performance. As we shall see, this has restricted studies of infant malnutrition; only recently have attempts been made to correlate the results of behavioral measurements made in infants below 2 years of age with tests performed at a later age.

In comparison to field studies of humans, animal models have several advantages. The diet can be closely controlled and frequently analyzed to ensure uniform composition. The environment can be regulated so that, except for the nutritional variable, conditions are nearly the same

128

for the experimental and control animals. Ethical considerations do not prevent the study of extreme or long-term effects and nutritional deprivation of various degrees can be maintained for prolonged periods. Perhaps the greatest advantage of using animal models is the opportunity to correlate behavioral changes with neurophysiologic changes and with histological, histochemical, and biochemical changes in the central nervous system.

One of the disadvantages of animal models is the difficulty in interpreting what a given behavior really means. For example, if an animal does not run a maze correctly is it because he is unable to learn the proper route or is it because he is not properly motivated to learn? Is he "hyperexcitable" and therefore unable to negotiate the maze? Is he ataxic and therefore unable to make tricky turns? All we can really say is that his performance in running a maze under the particular conditions of this experiment is impaired. Although this perhaps seems obvious, we shall see that many conclusions about "impaired learning ability" are based on these kinds of experiments.

Another problem in interpreting animal behavior derives from what was thought to be the chief advantage of using animals: the ability to control the environment except for the nutritional variable. While this may appear possible theoretically, in practice it has never been achieved. For example, producing malnutrition in neonatal rats by allowing 18 pups to suckle from a single mother certainly changes the pups' environment in ways other than simply restricting their food intake. Malnourishing the mother and having her nurse a normal-size litter does not solve this problem since a malnourished mother is apt to care for her pups quite differently from a well-nourished mother.

Since alterations of the neonatal environment, especially the interaction of mother and pups, will cause behavioral changes quite independent of the state of nutrition, the "pure neonatal malnutrition" experiment has not been done. Even with prenatal malnutrition, where this is less of a problem, maternal behavior may influence fetal development independent of maternal nutritional status.

Thus, neither animal nor human studies have been able to answer the crucial questions in this field fully. Does malnutrition per se during critical periods of development permanently alter behavior? If so, in what way? Is the ability to learn properly lost and, if so, is it a permanent loss? In this chapter I shall try to present what we have learned so far from both animal experiments and human studies.

ANIMAL STUDIES

Malnutrition and learning

Early research on rats was directed toward the effects of malnutrition on learning ability either during the period of malnutrition or after refeeding.[1, 2, 3, 4] The standard methods employed were all based on performance in one or another type of maze as a test of the animals' ability to learn. With the Hebb-Williams maze, for instance, the animal being tested was permitted only one trial after an initial period to familiarize itself with the chamber. The malnourished animals negotiated the maze less well than the well-fed animals. This inability to perform in the maze persisted to adulthood even if the animal was malnourished only for a brief period after birth. Because the use of only one trial was criticized as a poor test of learning, these experiments were repeated with multiple trials.[5] Again both the malnourished and the previously malnourished animals performed poorly.

A major criticism of both of these studies is that a food reward was used as an incentive for negotiating the maze.[6] Certainly malnourished animals will respond differently to such an incentive and this altered response to food may persist for long periods after the animal has been rehabilitated. Thus, it is impossible to conclude from these experiments that malnutrition early in life impairs learning.

In order to remove food as an incentive, other types of mazes that do not require a food incentive, such as water mazes, were employed.[7, 8] These studies were all based on some sort of stressful situation to initiate the animal to negotiate the maze. Again the malnourished and the previously malnourished animals did poorly, but again learning ability per se could not be implicated. Malnourished animals react differently to almost all types of stress and this altered response may in itself make the negotiation of the maze more difficult. Other types of studies to measure learning, like the standard bar-pressing experiment with all of its variations, have been employed. However, either a reward (usually food) or a punishment (usually electric shock) was used to "motivate learning," and the same criticism can be raised. The problem is that to measure the ability of an animal to learn you must get him to do something; what you actually measure is his ability to perform. This may or may not be impaired because of a learning deficit.

The early animal experiments on malnutrition, then, highlighted two areas of difficulty. The first was that although several types of behavior could be measured in a variety of animal species, the meaning of given behavioral changes was difficult to understand. The second was the isolation of malnutrition as the only variable. These are exactly the same two problems which face researchers studying the effects of malnutrition on subsequent behavior in human populations.

Malnutrition and "emotionality"

Classically, "emotionality" in rats has been tested by simply observing them in an open field. A rat is placed in a box with squares outlined on its floor. He is observed for a given period of time and the number of squares traversed (horizontal movement) as well as the number of times the animal rears up on his hind limbs (vertical movement) are recorded. The number of times the animal urinates and defecates is also recorded. Variations of this open field technique have also been employed in which a "novel stimulus" such as a rubber ball on a pendulum or a loud noise is introduced. The advantage of this experimental design is that the animal is neither rewarded nor punished but his natural behavior is simply observed.

When rats were malnourished during gestation and lactation, during lactation and for a period after weaning, or only during the post-weaning period, and then tested as adults, they showed decreased locomotor activity (horizontal movement), decreased rearing, head raising, and pivoting (vertical activity), and increased excretion of urine and feces. In addition, the adult rats remained at the periphery of the field, seldom venturing into the central squares.[1, 3, 9, 10, 11, 12, 13, 14, 15] This behavior has been interpreted as increased emotionality by some investigators and perhaps more accurately as decreased exploratory activity by others. All of the changes described could be markedly intensified by introducing a loud noise during the period of observation.[3, 5] Similar observations have been made in pigs tested in a modified open field after recovery from total food restriction or from a low-protein diet during the first 11 weeks of life.[16] Non-human primates fed a low-protein diet played significantly less, showed less sexual behavior, less grooming, and more aggressive behavior than animals that had been fed a high-protein diet.[17] Monkeys on a low-protein diet also showed less curiosity and puzzle-solving activity. It is interesting that as soon as a food reward was introduced these monkeys became more curious and solved puzzles as well as the controls. When the reward was withdrawn they returned to their apathetic state. In tests of social dominance the monkeys on a low-protein diet were submissive and always dominated by the control animals[18] (Fig. 5-1). Again, when food was introduced as a reward their behavior changed and they became more aggressive and domineering but returned to their passive state when the reward was no longer offered.

These studies have led investigators to conclude that the primary behavioral abnormality induced by early malnutrition is a breakdown in attention or observation. Many workers have shown that an appropriate observing response must develop in the monkey before he can learn to solve a discrimination problem.[17, 18, 19] It would appear that ani-

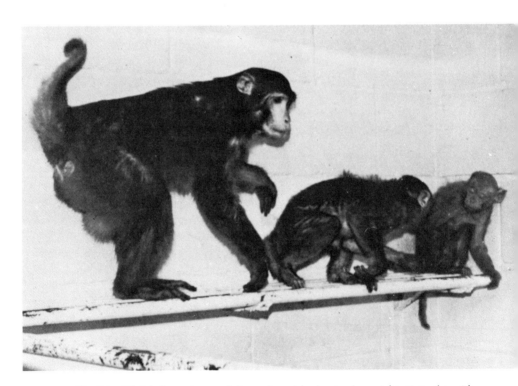

Fig. 5.1. Well-fed monkey on left—malnourished animal on right. Note the withdrawal of the malnourished animal who is dominated by the well-fed control.

mals subjected to a poor diet in early life do not develop this response adequately.

Whether this deficiency persists throughout life is not yet known for the primate. In the rat and pig similar deficiencies have been shown to persist. In human adults recovering from malnutrition attention span improves as the preoccupation with food declines. On the other hand, similar behavioral abnormalities have been shown to persist in infants who have recovered from previous malnutrition.

Malnutrition and other behaviors

The development of certain reflexes (i.e. startle, grasp, visual placing) and certain physical characteristics (eye opening, incisor eruption) is delayed in malnourished animals. This retardation will naturally result in delayed development of behavior that depends on the maturation of these reflexes and physical characteristics, and it is assuming more and more importance in our understanding of the behavioral consequences of early malnutrition. The developmental process is one of continuing interaction between an organism and his environment at critical times. If the timing of this interaction is disturbed, profound behavioral abnormalities may occur. Thus if an animal cannot receive visual stimuli at the proper time because his eyes have not yet opened his entire subsequent development may be altered. This concept extends not only to alterations in the appearance of physical abilities necessary to receive environmental stimuli but also to the institution of behavioral changes such as those just described in motivation and attention which in turn preclude proper integration of necessary environmental input. Thus, those holding this view on the mechanism by which malnutrition alters behavior would argue that there are three elements involved in determining behavior: the infant, the environment, and the time at which these two interact.

The early environment and behavior

A large body of literature, which we will only touch on, demonstrates that in a variety of animal species profound behavioral changes will occur if the early environment is disturbed. Moreover, many of these changes persist into adult life. A "stimulatory environment" for rats has been created by frequent handling of the animals during early life, by electric shock, and by exposure to brief periods of cold from birth to 21 days of age.[20] A severely deprived environment has been produced by rearing rats in the dark in a sound-proof room and in single cages. Less severe deprivation has been applied to monkeys by isolating the young from the mother and feeding them by simply placing a bottle in the cage.

Stimulation of well-nourished rats decreases emotionality, increases exploratory behavior, and decreases reactions to adverse stimuli. Isolation of well-nourished rats causes the reverse. Thus the well-nourished but isolated rat shows behavioral characteristics quite similar to the rat malnourished in early life. Isolation of monkeys produces a bizzare behavioral pattern which includes apathy, decreased exploratory behavior, withdrawal from the environment, and heightened emotional responses when confronted with stress. Again we see behavior in the well-fed isolated animals that is similar to the behavior of animals that were poorly fed in early life.

This similarity between the effects of early malnutrition and early isolation becomes even more striking if certain physiological and biochemical data are examined. In rats, isolation will reduce the rate of cell division, the rate of myelination and the number of dendritic arborizations and will elevate the activity of acetylcholinesterase. Stimulation produces the reverse. The biochemical changes associated with isolation are like those found in the brains of animals subjected to early malnutrition. This suggests not only that there is an obvious need for strict environmental control in experiments on malnutrition, but also that environmental deprivation and malnutrition may interact during the early postnatal period.

One approach to producing early malnutrition in the rat, as we have seen, has been to increase litter size during lactation. By increasing litter size, however, one not only reduces the amount of milk for each pup but also increases the amount of sibling stimulation and decreases the amount of attention given by the dam to each pup.[21] Exploring this problem, Frankova reported that there is considerable behavioral difference among pups from litters of different size. Exploratory behavior and spontaneous activity in the open field proved to be greatest in intermediate litter sizes (9 to 13 pups), less in the smallest (4 pups), and lowest in the largest litters (17 pups). There was also an inverse relationship between body weight and litter size (the smallest body weights were found in the largest litters). Frankova concluded that it is the interaction between sibling stimulation and neonatal nutrition that determines exploratory behavior and "emotionality" in the adult.

Levitsky and Barnes have given this hypothesis further support in experiments with rats that were either well nourished or protein malnourished for seven weeks and were then subjected to environmental stimulation, isolation, or normal social conditions.[22] Behavioral testing after refeeding revealed a highly significant interaction between isolation and early malnutrition with regard to locomotor activity and exploratory behavior. The isolated malnourished group showed much less of both than either the well-nourished or the other malnourished group. Environmental stimulation seemed to compensate for early malnutrition as the stimulated malnourished group was rated very close to all of the well-nourished animals in locomotor and exploratory behavior. Cines and her colleagues have reported similar results with stimulated and non-stimulated rats undernourished for the first 3 weeks of life and subsequently rehabilitated.[23] Studying the same rats, Coombs and his colleagues reported that the biochemical abnormalities of the brain usually produced by neonatal undernutrition did not fully appear when stimulation was introduced.[24] The protein/DNA ratio, the RNA/DNA ratio, and the activity of alkaline RNase all approached normal in the stimulated malnourished animals, but DNA content (cell number) was still reduced. These studies demonstrate that some of the effects of malnutrition on development of the central nervous system of the rat can be reversed by enriching the animal's early environment.

Recently, Frankova has attempted a new means of increasing stimulation: introducing a trained virgin female as an "aunt" into the cage with the mother and pups from 8 a.m. to 4 p.m.[25] The aunt assists the mother in caring for the pups, retrieves them, grooms them, and generally provides a heightened level of stimulation. The result was an increased interaction between individual pups and more interaction between the pups and their mother when the aunt was present. This form of stimulation changes the mother's as well as the pups' behavior, and the improvement was more marked in malnourished than well-fed animals. These studies provide the first clearcut proof that environment and nutritional state interact in determining behavior in the adult animal.

What is the nature of this interaction between environment and malnutrition in the first few weeks of life that influences the final behavioral repertoire of the adult animal? Levitsky and Barnes have suggested that malnutrition, by producing apathy and decreased curiosity, may make the animal less susceptible to environmental programming.[5] Malnutrition may therefore indirectly prevent the proper stimulus from arriving at the proper time and, since experience is cumulative the animal unable to build on previous experience would be retarded in his development. Malnutrition reduces the range and amount of information available to the developing animal. Having been exposed to fewer earlier experiences the adult animal is limited in its ability to cope with a normal variety of environmental stimuli. This limitation may in turn inhibit the processes of mental development and socialization.

It should be pointed out that although this explanation which proposes a "final common pathway," isolation from the environment, as the actual cause of the behavioral abnormalities seen in malnutrition is attractive it is not necessarily correct. An alternative explanation is possible if one postulates that the brain has a limited number of responses which it makes to alterations in the environment. Thus malnutrition and isolation may affect the brain quite independently and through different mechanisms. The response however is similar and the behavioral manifestations of that response indistinguishable.

Regardless of the explanation, however, it is encouraging that preliminary evidence suggests that enriching the environment does have redeeming effects in the malnourished animal. The obvious clinical relevance of this finding makes confirmation of these findings imperative.

In general then it can be said that the animal experiments have not proven an association between early malnutrition and learning. They have shown that animals malnourished in a variety of ways both prenatally and postnatally show behavioral abnormalities best described as increased emotionality and decreased exploratory activity. This behavioral pattern persists even after rehabilitation. Similar behavioral abnormalities have been induced in young animals by isolating them from their environment and partial reversal of the effects of malnutrition is possible if the environment is enriched. After more than two decades of experiments the basic problems are still present. The animal experiments have certainly not solved the question of early malnutrition and later mental development, nor in my opinion can they ever solve this problem until the actual biochemical and neurophysiological mechanisms controlling specific behaviors are understood and the effects of malnutrition on these mechanisms studied. Thus the importance of animal behavior work in the future will be directly proportional to its use in deriving a better understanding of the basic mechanisms controlling behavior. As part of this approach, the effects of early malnutrition may be better understood but perhaps more importantly early malnutrition may provide a useful experimental model by which this mechanistic approach can be facilitated.

HUMAN STUDIES

Investigators in several countries have tried to examine the effects of malnutrition early in life on subsequent human behavior. Most of these studies have focused on measuring intelligence because testing procedures are readily available and because the demonstration of persistent intellectual deficits would have immediate social impact. Rather than attempting to review all such studies I will group them into several categories and discuss representative studies in each category in detail.

Early malnutrition and intelligence

Malnutrition in deprived populations

The intellectual development of children severely malnourished as infants has been studied both retrospectively[26, 27, 28, 29] and prospectively.[30, 31, 32, 33] In both types of studies, however, it is difficult to isolate malnutrition as the cause of any mental deficiencies found, since the malnourished children invariably come from a lower socio-economic class and a generally more deprived environment than even the most carefully matched control groups. Both types of studies also suffer from the lack of standardization of intelligence tests. It has been pointed out many times before that tests developed in industrialized nations may have little meaning in developing countries with very different cultures.

In addition, with retrospective studies one can never be sure of the criteria used to establish the diagnosis of malnutrition or of what other social factors may have affected the development of the malnourished children.

In a retrospective analysis, Cabak and Najdanvic demonstrated that Serbian children with a history of marasmus had significantly lower intelligence quotients than Serbian children in general.[26] They made no real attempt to control other environmental factors but selected individuals of the same racial or genetic stock for comparison. One important aspect of this study is that it deals with malnutrition during the first year of life. Precise time distinctions are often not made in such studies. Compared to other investigations the Cabak and Najdanvic study showed one of the largest intelligence quotient deficits and its subjects were the youngest when nutritionally deprived. The major weakness of the study was the lack of an adequate control group. The children selected for comparison not only were better nourished but came from higher socio-economic strata.

Retrospective studies in developing countries throughout the world in which better control groups have been chosen do suggest that early malnutrition interferes with subsequent learning ability. In a study of 107 Indonesian children between 12 and 15 years of age from lower socio-economic groups, including 46 who had been previously classified as malnourished, the Wechsler Intelligence Scale for Children and Goodenough tests were used.[34] The better nourished, taller children scored higher than the previously malnourished, shorter children. The lowest I.Q.s were associated with the poorest prior nutritional status. At the Nutrition Research Laboratories in Hyderabad, India, a rather thorough study was conducted to determine whether school children treated for kwashiorkor some years before were retarded in comparison to other children attending the same school.[35] Nineteen children who had been treated for kwashiorkor between 1959 and 1962, and who were 8 to 11 years of age at the time of follow-up, were studied. The records showed that the children had been admitted to hospital at ages ranging from 1.5 to 3.0 years and that a diagnosis of kwashiorkor had been made in each case. As a control group 3 "matched" children were chosen for each child under study. They were matched for age, sex, religion, caste, socio-economic status, family size, and educational background of the parents, and they were in the same school class and came from the same locality as the children being studied.

Such careful matching might be expected to influence the study against demonstrating differences between the two groups. Children subjected to severe malnutrition frequently do not survive. If they live, they may not go to school; and if they attend school, they may be in a grade below that which is normal for their age. The results of the Indian study, however, still showed significant behavioral differences.

The intelligence tests, standardized in India, included items to test different mental functions such as reasoning, organization of knowledge, memory, and different perceptual processes. Reading comprehension and arithmetic tests were used to measure the children's ability to do abstract reasoning. Perceptual ability was tested by picture completion and simplified object assembly and block design.[36] Intersensory organization and neurointegrative development were also measured, using standardized tests for these functions.

Differences in the test scores were greatest in the younger children (aged 8-9 years). The previously malnourished children were more retarded in their perceptual and abstracting ability than in their memory and verbal ability. Their performance was also poorer in the intersensory tests, particularly the visual-haptic test. The previously malnourished children were smaller and lighter than the controls in every age group, but their head circumferences were not significantly different.

The test score differences in this study are greater than those reported in other studies (about a 35 point I.Q. difference), and these differences exist six or more years after clinical recovery from kwashiorkor.

While it is tempting to conclude that kwashiorkor, and the protein deficient diet that preceded it, caused the poor mental performance of the Indian children who had the disease, other factors may have been involved. All 19 children had been treated in the hospital for a period of at least 6 weeks and many probably were either bed-ridden or relatively inactive for long periods of time before and after the episode of the serious illness. This prolonged period of relative immobilization could have resulted in a loss of "learning time," while the stress of separation from home and family during hospitalization might possibly have had a long-term effect. Among the uncontrolled variables in the study were the motivation and responsiveness of the parents, educational levels of the parents, child spacing, and infectious diseases. The authors themselves conclude that "although the differences in mental performance between the two groups of children investigated in this study are clearcut, it is not easy at this stage to determine to what extent this is a result of the episode of kwashiorkor and to what extent it is due to other factors."

More recently, Chase has reported that infants in the United States who were severely malnourished early in life performed consistently poorly when later tested.[27] Though his study does not isolate malnutrition as the only important variable, it does make clear that the complex of social problems and nutritional deprivation operating in developing countries is prevalent among certain groups in our own country and is associated with the same type of retarded development.

A number of prospective studies of malnutrition and mental development have been done or are currently under way. Stoch and Smythe, studying South African children, have shown that those malnourished early in life are smaller than a control population and have reduced head circumferences and intelligence quotients even after long-term follow-up. The intelligence quotient testing was adapted for South African children and would appear to be valid. Again, however, the control population leaves much to be desired. The malnourished children lived in inadequate housing with no sanitary facilities, came from poverty-stricken and often broken homes, and were generally neglected. Control families chosen from an industry-built project lived in neat brick houses which had sanitary facilities; all the fathers and mothers were employed and all the children had attended nursery school.

The problem of finding an adequate control population is not easily solved by matching socio-economic backgrounds. In a Jamaican study Garrett and Pike used siblings without a history of hospitalization for malnutrition as a control group for those who had such a history and found that the malnourished group reached the same height and weight and I.Q. score as the control group.[28] Here we see the opposite problem. In this study, the control children probably were also malnourished, sub-clinically if not clinically. Both groups of children had poor growth and development compared to generally accepted Jamaican norms and significantly retarded growth by United States standards. In a more extensive study carried out recently in Jamaica, 74 male children who had been hospitalized for severe malnutrition before they were two years of age were compared with their closest aged brothers and classmates.[37] All the children were between 6 and 11 years of age when studied. Neurological status, intersensory competence, intellectual level, and a variety of language, perceptual, and motor abilities were evaluated. Intellectual level was significantly lower in the index cases than in their brothers or classmates. As might be expected, the classmate comparison group did best and the index cases worst, with the siblings between. The difference in the brothers' and classmates' scores again points out a disadvantage of studies employing only siblings as controls: the presence of one child hospitalized for severe malnutrition might be expected to identify a high-risk family for chronic undernutrition. This may be important from the standpoint of rapid case finding. Identification of a severely malnourished infant should alert the therapist to examine all of the siblings in the family.

Why one sibling in a family develops severe malnutrition and others do not is a perplexing question, though the assumption that all children in a family have equal access to food and maternal care, and have similar experiences in the home, clearly is not always correct. It could be that one child was not wanted, or was born during a period of family crisis, and thus was deprived of food and parental attention. Sometimes one sibling is relatively neglected because he or she is less attractive to the mother. Child-rearing practices within a family change, with varying nutrition and parental stimulation for each sibling.

One of the best series of nutrition studies to date is that of Cravioto and others in Mexico and Guatemala.[30, 31, 32] In populations of uniform socio-economic backgrounds, performance on psychological tests was found to be related to dietary practice and not to differences in personal hygiene, housing, cash income, crop income, proportion of income spent on food, parental education, or other social or economic indicators. Moreover, performance of both preschool and school children on the Terman, Merrill, Gesell, and Goodenough Draw-A-Man tests was positively correlated with body weights and heights. These tests had been adapted for the population studied. Further investigations in collaboration with the Institute of Nutrition of Central America and Panama (INCAP) in Guatemala again showed a positive correlation between size and performance. The tests included placing blocks in openings, tracing block shapes, and differentiating block shapes by touch alone. These tasks were considered to be measures of visual, haptic, and kinesthetic sensory integration, respectively. To confirm that the differences in height reflected differences in previous nutrition and not familial tendencies, the child's height was correlated with the height of his parents. This correlation proved to be extremely poor, a sharp contrast to the significant correlation in affluent populations between the height of children and that of their parents. (In populations where malnutrition is not prevalent it is also true that short children perform as well as tall children on tests such as those used in the INCAP studies.) Since the shorter children they studied did not come from families significantly lower in socio-economic status, housing, and parental education than those of the taller children, Cravioto and his associates concluded that the most important variable reflected by the short stature was poor nutrition during early life and that this also led to the lag in development of sensory integrative competence.

A number of other studies have expanded on these observations. Examining another aspect of neurointegrative competence and auditory and visual integration in Mexican children of school age from communities where malnutrition is common, Cravioto, Espinosa, and Birch found that the taller children could integrate information received from both stimuli better than the shorter children of the same age.[38] This observation is particularly important since integrative ability is essential in acquiring primary reading skills. A major consideration in interpreting the findings of this and other studies is the fact that antecedent malnutrition is being inferred from differences in height rather than by direct observation of dietary intake during the growing years. Much evidence suggests that this interpretation is valid. Observations by Boas on growth differences in successive generations of the American-born children of Jewish immigrants, of Boyd-Orr on secular trends in the height of British children, of Grulich on the height of Japanese immigrants, of Mitchell on the relation of nutrition to stature, of Buderkeun-Young on Italian children, as well as the recent study of heights of twelve-year-old Puerto Rican boys in New York City by Abromovitz all support the inference. It is significant that in the study made by Cravioto and his associates in Mexico, the earlier the malnutrition, the more profound the psychological retardation. The most severe retardation occurred in children admitted to the hospital under 6 months of age and did not improve on serial testing even after 220 days of treatment. Children admitted later in life with the same socio-economic background and the same severe malnutrition did recover after prolonged rehabilitation. This recovery of older children even when severely malnourished has been observed before. Kuglemaus and associates found retardation in a group of malnourished children over 6 years of age; with prolonged rehabilitation the children significantly increased their intelligence quotient scores.

Although it has been shown that early malnutrition is more likely to produce lasting effects than malnutrition occurring later in life, the exact time span when malnutrition has the most serious effect is not yet known. In the Jamaican study mentioned above, for example, Birch and his associates found that in all of the children malnourished at any time during the first 2 years of life significant behavioral abnormalities persisted at school age. Moreover, the severity of these functional difficulties did not differ with the time during the first 2 years of life that the malnutrition occurred. On the surface the results of this study would seem to differ from the results of the studies by Cravioto et al., in which children under 6 months of age recovered less well than children malnourished after reaching 6 months of age. Closer examination of the two studies can probably explain the differences. In the Mexican study the children were followed only until 22 months of age whereas in the Jamaican study they were examined 6 to 10 years later. The results of the two studies are compatible if one assumes that malnutrition during the first 6 months of life requires a longer period of rehabilitation for the children to achieve their maximum functional potential than malnutrition occurring later in the first 2 years of life. This presumes that both groups of children ultimately are able to recover to the same point, but that point would appear to be at a lower level of functioning than children who had never been malnourished.

Malnutrition in more affluent populations

In nearly all research on humans to date, the malnourished subjects (and sometimes the control children) have come from the lower socio-economic stratum of a population. The need to study malnourished children who were not raised in a deprived environment has not been adequately recognized, though it has been suggested that the survivors of severe famines and of conditions such as celiac disease should be studied.[39] Only very recently have the first reports of such studies become available.

The 1944-45 famine in the Netherlands was sharply circumscribed in place and time, the nutritional deprivation was well documented, and extensive data were available for subsequent analysis. For 6 months 750 or fewer calories were available per person each day in the famine area of western Holland, whereas food rations provided at least (and often much more) than 1300 calories per person per day in the non-famine areas in the rest of Holland. In the famine areas death rates from starvation were high, famine edema was prevalent, and many subjects lost 25% or more of their original body weight.

A retrospective cohort study of male inductees into the armed forces from both areas of Holland was recently undertaken.[40] Those born between early 1944 and the end of 1946 were divided into separate cohorts according to whether they were conceived or born before, during, or after the famine.

Among these groups of survivors the frequency of severe or mild mental retardation (International Classification of Diseases 3250, 3251, 3252, and 3254) was not related to conception, pregnancy, or birth during the famine. Test scores of several thousand young men on the Dutch version of the Raven progressive matrices showed no differences between those coming from famine and non-famine areas when they were medically examined at the time of induction into the armed services. The intelligence tests which failed to show differences between famine and non-famine subjects were sufficiently sensitive to show highly significant differences in rates of mental retardation between inductees of two social classes, namely manual and non-manual workers. Thus, although no effect on mental development could be detected, a very significant association between the social class of the father and both mental retardation and intelligence test scores was found. It was also found that birth weights in the famine areas were significantly lower than in the non-famine areas of Holland and that a decline in fertility affected the manual workers more than the non-manual workers.

The conclusions of this study differ markedly from research findings in most other countries. It has already been stressed, however, that the malnourished children in all previous investigations suffered many deprivations other than nutritional deficiencies. The Dutch were generally well nourished before the famine occurred. After the famine dietary and other serious deprivations were relatively uncommon in their country. The Dutch research suggests that if there is an impairment in fetal development due to maternal starvation, it is not of a degree that cannot be overcome by standard child-rearing practices as they exist in Holland. A second interpretation, based on the high mortality in the famine years, is that infants who would have been severely retarded died. This interpretation postulates an "all or none" response which is unlikely.

Children with cystic fibrosis represent another nutritionally deprived population that is more or less free of socio-economic deprivation. The disease is characterized by chronic pancreatic insufficiency, fatty diarrhea, and chronic lung disease. Malnutrition occurs very early in life due to malabsorption of nutrients. A study was made of middle-class children with cystic fibrosis who suffered prolonged malnutrition during their first 6 months of life, with weights below the third percentile on the Boston (Stuart) growth charts for at least 4 of those first 6 months.[41] All the children had other evidence of severe malnutrition resembling the symptoms of kwashiorkor or marasmus. Twenty-nine siblings of these malnourished children served as controls, and I.Q. tests were given to 27 of the parents.

The malnourished children who were under 5 years of age showed lower scores on the Merrill Palmer tests than the control children. There were no significant differences between the scores of study and control children over five on the Wechsler Intelligence Scale for Children (WISC), the Vineland Scale of Social Maturity or the Wechsler Adult

Intelligence Scale (which was given to those children over 14 years of age at the end of the study).

The results seem to show that malnutrition in the early months of life is associated with poorer scores on psychological tests while a child is ill and during the early years of life immediately following, or during recovery from malnutrition. Differences in I.Q. apparently disappear after 5 years of age.

The studies on non-deprived populations strongly suggest that early malnutrition may retard development temporarily but that recovery is possible given the proper subsequent environment. These conclusions underline the importance of two other types of investigations currently being carried out: serial studies of the effects of malnutrition on mental development and studies which attempt to enrich the environment of children who have been malnourished as infants.

Serial studies on intellectual development of malnourished children

Serial studies of intellectual development will allow observations of the time when recovery from malnutrition occurs and the conditions necessary to facilitate recovery. The major obstruction to these studies is the difficulty in structuring "psychometric tests" for infants and young children which can predict later intelligence. Only a few such tests are useful with normal children and none has had careful trials with malnourished children. Recently, however, Klein and his associates at INCAP have attempted to evaluate the usefulness of an "orienting response" in predicting later intellectual deficits in malnourished children.[42] In a preliminary study these investigators presented 40 trials of a pure tone auditory stimulus to 8 marginally nourished and 8 malnourished 13½-month-old male infants. Initially, the marginally malnourished children had a greater orientation response (as measured by a slowing of their heart beat) than the malnourished children. When the stimulus tone was changed the marginally nourished children again showed a greater response. The authors cite evidence that the lower response seen in the malnourished children is a sign of poor attention which in other children tested by this method led to poor learning later on. Whether this will prove to be true in malnourished children is still unknown, but follow-up studies of this population should answer the question.

Environmental enrichment for malnourished children

Several studies have indicated that enriching the environment in deprived populations of children can improve their subsequent development.[43, 44, 45] Generally children from a low socio-economic class have been randomly assigned to either a treatment or a control group. The treatment group receives a variety of special care and instruction through home visits and day-care-center experience. The results in general have shown that the "stimulated children" develop better and show a higher I.Q. at the end of the experience. Unfortunately after most of these studies have ended the child has been "returned" to his normal environment and his I.Q. usually reverts to the level of the control group.

One study in which long-term stimulation was applied is noteworthy.[46] Two groups of mentally retarded, institutionalized children whose mothers' average I.Q. was under 70 were studied. Thirteen of these children were transferred at age two from an orphanage to a state institution for the mentally retarded. The children were placed in the care of older female inmates in a one to one mother child relationship. After one and a half years these children had gained 28 I.Q. points whereas the children left at the orphanage had lost 26 I.Q. points. After two and a half years of legal adoption the study children reached a mean I.Q. of 101. These children were followed up thirty years later. They were self-supporting and most had completed twelfth grade. Four of the children had one or more years of college. By contrast, most of the children left at the orphanage had completed only third grade and were at institutions for the mentally retarded. In addition, a number of them had died.

In order to examine the effects of "environmental enrichment" on the development of malnourished children, two studies are currently under way. One is a retrospective analysis of a population of Korean children, some of whom were severely malnourished during the first year of life and were then adopted by families in the United States.[47] The second is a prospective study in Colombia where malnourished infants are identified in the hospital and then placed in a special nursery school environment at two years of age.[48]

We have studied 141 Korean girls, dividing them into three groups. Forty-two were severely malnourished, below the third percentile for both height and weight when compared to Korean standards. Fifty-two were marginally nourished, between the third and twenty-fifth percentile for height and weight, and 47 were well nourished, above the fiftieth percentile for height and weight. Only infants falling into these categories before their first birthdays were selected. All of the infants were adopted before their second birthday by American families. The adoptions were entirely random on a first come, first served basis. The parents had no idea of a child's previous nutritional history. All of the families were carefully screened to ensure an adequate home environment for the adopted child. Questionnaires were sent to all of the families and records were obtained from the schools the children were attending. Their ages at the time of follow-up ranged from 7 to 16 years. Intelligence tests were administered by the schools. Achievement based on a number of other test scores which were available was evaluated by two psychologists having no prior knowledge of the children's history.

By the time these children reached seven years of age there were no differences in average weight among the three groups (Fig. 5-2). All had reached normal by Korean standards but were significantly below normal by American standards. Changes in height were similar to those in weight except that the malnourished children remained slightly but

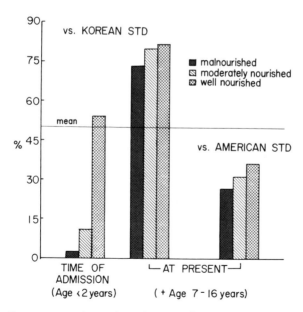

Fig. 5.2. Changes in weight in adopted Korean children

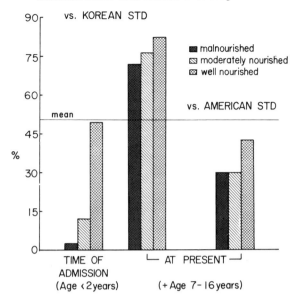

Fig. 5.3.   Changes in height in adopted Korean children

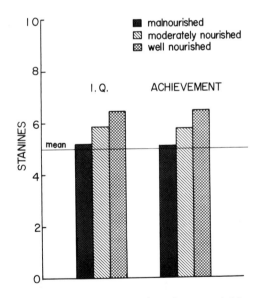

Fig. 5.4.   Intelligence and achievement in adopted Korean children

significantly smaller (Fig. 5-3). The mean I.Q. of the previously malnourished group was 102.05. The marginally nourished children achieved a mean I.Q. of 105.95. This is not a statistically significant difference. By contrast, the previously well-nourished children reached a mean I.Q. of 111.68, which does represent a significant difference from the malnourished children. When achievement in these three groups was compared, the results were similar. Both the severely malnourished and the marginally malnourished children were achieving exactly at expected norms for American children of the same age and the same grade (Fig. 5-4). The previously well-nourished children were achieving slightly but significantly better.

These findings show that severely malnourished children, when reared in a middle-class environment, can catch up in height and weight and reach an I.Q. and school achievement level which is perfectly normal for well-nourished children raised in an industrialized nation. They demonstrate in this unique population exactly what has been shown in animal studies, that environmental stimulation will reverse many if not all of the behavioral deficits elicited by early malnutrition. The data also suggest that when well-nourished children are placed in this more stimulating environment they do even better. Their I.Q. scores and achievement scores are not only higher than those of the malnourished children but also are higher than the norms for American children in general. From a practical standpoint the importance of this study lies in its pointing out the reversibility of effects of early malnutrition. In all previous studies when the child was returned to his or her previous environment the I.Q. was 70 or below at school age (Table 5-1).

In the previous studies when children were reared in a poor socioeconomic environment even those who were adequately nourished and used as controls reached a maximum I.Q. of 82. The malnourished children average about 10 points lower. Thus the difference between the malnourished and the well-nourished children is similar in this study to the previous studies. All of the children simply do better.

In the prospective study in Colombia, severely malnourished children after recovery have been placed in an "enriched" environment at about two years of age.[48] The children are exposed to all types of stimulating experiences in terms of both play and learning. Their nutrition has been kept adequate. These children are being compared with randomly picked similarly malnourished children who were not placed in this program and with previously well-nourished children of higher socio-economic

Table 5-1
SELECTED I.Q. STUDIES OF CHILDREN
MALNOURISHED BETWEEN 2-3 YEARS OF AGE

Author	Sex	N.*	Mean I.Q.	S.D.	T.	P.	Follow up age (yrs.)
Stoch & Smyth	Mixed	I=21	61.15	8.08	6.06	0.01	10-13
(1963) S. Africa		C=21	77.50	9.35			
Birch et. al.	Fems.	I=23	68.6	13.83	1.05	N.S.	5-13
(1971) Mexico		C=16	72.8	10.92			
	Males	I=14	70.7	14.08	1.07	0.05	
		C=21	82.3	16.12			
Hertzig, Birch		I=71	57.72	10.75	5.25	0.01	6-10
et. al. (1972)	Males	S=38	61.84	10.82	2.08	0.025	
Jamaica		C=71	65.99	13.59	1.83	0.01	
Winick, Meyer,		I=37[+]	102.05	10.16	1.45	N.S.	7-16
Harris, et. al.	Fems.	II=38[+]	105.95	12.88	3.49	0.01	
(1975) U.S.A.		C=37[+]	111.68	13.27	1.89	0.06	

I = Index or Group I
S = Siblings—moderately or chronically malnourished
II = Group II—moderately or chronically malnourished
C = Controls—well nourished
Numbers vary because of inadequate data.

class both in and out of the program. Preliminary results suggest that stimulation will improve the learning of these children. The test levels of the stimulated malnourished children were higher than those of the non-stimulated malnourished children and approached those of the children from the higher socio-economic group who were not stimulated. The well-nourished, stimulated children had the highest learning capacity but as the study progresses their lead is shortening.

Dietary supplementation

A final group of studies, of human populations, has focused on improvement in the nutrition of pregnant women and young infants. The basic design of these studies involves comparing a population undergoing severe malnutrition with a similar population that is given nutritional supplements. After a given period of time the results are evaluated in terms of whatever outcome measures the investigators choose. Not only are such studies technically difficult to carry out but they also involve ethical problems, especially with regard to the non-intervention groups. For these reasons only a few have been carried out and these under conditions and in populations that have been carefully selected. One study is being done by INCAP in three rural Guatemalan villages.[49] Great pains have been taken to ensure that these villages have comparable populations. One village receives a food supplement in the form of a high-protein supplement drink that is consumed by the young children and the pregnant mothers. A second village is supplied with a supplement of some caloric value but no protein content. Both villages are given medical care. The third village receives medical care only. Preliminary results show that growth rates are increased in the children receiving the high-protein supplement. Moreover, the women who get a protein supplement during pregnancy have babies whose birth weight is significantly higher than that of babies born in the non-supplemented village (Fig. 5-5). Finally it would appear that the development of the children is better in the protein supplemented village than in the other villages.

In a second study in Formosa, supplementation of mothers' diets after they have had a baby and throughout their next pregnancy has significantly increased the birth weight of the second infant.[50] In a third study

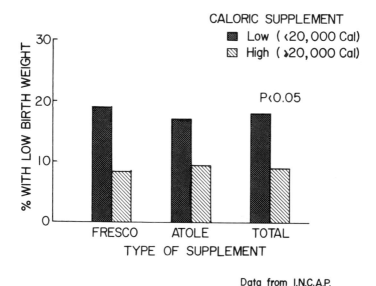

Fig. 5.5. Effect of protein (Atole) and caloric (Fresco) supplementation on birth weight

in the United States, supplementation of the diets of pregnant women from a poor urban population has resulted in an increased birth weight of their babies.[51] In a small study in rural Mexico food supplements have been given to children of families carefully selected to represent the norms of their community.[52] When the growth rate of the supplemented children was compared with that of their previously studied, unsupplemented siblings a marked increase was observed. The supplemented children also demonstrated marked superiority in physical strength, independence, attentiveness, and ability to perform certain behavioral tests. They tended to explore their environment more thoroughly, play with toys more frequently and interact with adults better than the non-supplemented children. It must be emphasized that the children in this study who did not receive the supplement were picked because they were representative of the village and not because they were malnourished.

The sparse information that is available from intervention studies, then, would suggest that improvement in the diet during either pregnancy or early life will significantly alter birth weight, subsequent growth rate, and subsequent behavior.

These studies have begun to elicit a response on the part of governments to re-examine their priorities in the area of nutrition in vulnerable groups. Some governments, including our own, have instituted specific programs designed to improve nutrition in pregnant women and young infants. Most of these programs are in the "demonstration" stage. It is extremely important that they be carefully monitored so that information on their success or failure will be forthcoming. At present, this is not being done.

REFERENCES

1. Cowley, J. J., and Griesel, R. D. Some effects of a low-protein diet on a first filial generation of white rats, J. Genet. Psychol. 95:187, 1959.
2. Cowley, J. J., and Griesel, R. D. The development of a second generation of low-protein rats, J. Genet. Psychol. 103:233, 1963.
3. Cowley, J. J., and Griesel, R. D. Low-protein diet and emotionality in the albino rat, J. Genet. Psychol. 104:89, 1964.
4. Cowley, J. J., and Griesel, R. D. The effect on growth and behavior of rehabilitating first and second generation low-protein rats, Animal Behavior 14:506, 1966.

5. Levitsky, D. A., and Barnes, R. H. Effect of early malnutrition on reaction of adult rats to adverse stimuli, Nature 225:468, 1970.

6. Barnes, R. H. Reported at Gordon Research Conf., New London, N.H., August 1967.

7. Barnes, R. H., Cunnold, S. R., Zimmerman, R. R., Simmons, H., Mac Leod, R. B., and Krook, L. Influence of nutritional deprivations in early life on learning behavior of rats as measured by performance in a water maze, J. Nutr. 89:399, 1966.

8. Kerr, G. R., and Waisman, H. A. Cited in.Feeding and Nutrition of Non-Human Primates, Harris, R. S., ed., New York, Academic Press, 1970.

9. Simonson, M., Stephen, J. K., Hanson, H. M., and Chow, B. F. Open field studies in offspring of underfed mother rats, J. Nutr. 101:331, 1971.

10. Lat, J., Widdowson, E. M., and McCance, R. A. Some effects of accelerating growth. III. Behavior and nervous activity, Proc. R. Soc., Biol., Ser. B, 153:347, 1961.

11. Altman, J., Sudarsham, K., Das, G. D., McCormick, N., and Barnes, D. The influence of nutrition on neural and behavioral development. III. Development of some motor, particularly locomotor patterns during infancy, Devel. Psychobiol. 4:97, 1971.

12. Levitsky, D. A., and Barnes, R. H. Effect of early malnutrition on reaction of adult rats to adverse stimuli, Nature 225:468, 1970.

13. Frankova, S., and Barnes, R. H. Influence of malnutrition in early life on exploratory behavior of rats, J. Nutr. 96:477, 1968.

14. Guthrie, H. A. Severe undernutrition in early infancy and behavior in rehabilitated albino rats, Physiol. Behav. 3:619, 1968.

15. Barnett, S. A., Smart, J. L., and Widdowson, E. M. Early nutrition and the activity and feeding of rats in an artificial environment, Develop. Psychobiol. 4:1, 1971.

16. Barnes, R. H., Moore, A. V., and Pond, W. G. Behavioral abnormalities in young adult pigs caused by malnutrition in early life, J. Nutr. 100:149, 1970.

17. Zimmermann, R. R., Steere, P. O., Strobel, D. A., and Hom, H. L. Abnormal social development of protein malnourished rhesus monkeys, J. Abnormal Psychol. 80:125, 1972.

18. Wise, L. A. The effects of protein deprivation on dominance measured by shock avoidance competition and food competition, unpublished masters' thesis, University of Montana.

19. Strobel, D. A., and Zimmermann, R. R. Manipulatory responsiveness in protein malnourished monkeys, Psychon. Sci. 24:19, 1971.

20. Levine, S., and Denenberg, V. Separate reviews, in Stimulation in Early Infancy, Ambrose, A., ed., London, Academic Press, 1969, p. 21.

21. Seitz, P. F. D. The effects of infantile experiences upon adult behavior in animal subjects: I. Effects of litter size during infancy upon adult behavior in the rat, Am. J. Psychiat. 110:916, 1954.

22. Levitsky, D. A., and Barnes, R. H. Nutritional and environmental inter-

actions in the behavioral development of the rat: Long-term effects, Science 176:68, 1972.

23. Cines, B. Reported at Symposium on Nutrition and Fetal Development presented by the Institute of Human Nutrition and sponsored by the National Foundation-March of Dimes, New York City, 1972.

24. Coombs, J. Personal communication.

25. Frankova, S. Interaction between early malnutrition and stimulation in animals, in Symposia of the Swedish Nutrition Foundation XII, Early Malnutrition and Mental Development, Cravioto, J., Hambraeus, L., and Vahlquist, B., eds., Uppsala, Almqvist & Wiksell, 1974, p. 226.

26. Cabak, V., and Najdanvic, R. Effect of undernutrition in early life on physical and mental development, Arch. Dis. Child. 40:532, 1965.

27. Chase, H. P. Presented to the Society for Pediatric Research, Atlantic City, N.J., 1969.

28. Garrow, J. S., and Pike, M. C. The long-term prognosis of severe malnutrition, Lancet 1:1, 1967.

29. Graham, G. G. The effect of infantile malnutrition on growth, Fed. Proc. 26:139, 1967.

30. Cravioto, J., and Robles, B. Evolution of adaptive and motor behavior during rehabilitation from kwashiorkor, Amer. J. Orthopsychiat. 35:449, 1965.

31. Cravioto, J., Birch, H. G., and DeLicardie, E. R. Influencia de la desnutricion en la capacidad de apprendizajo del nino escolar, Bol. Med. Hosp. Infantil., Mexico 24:217, 1967.

32. Cravioto, J., DeLicardie, E. R., and Birch, H. G. Nutrition, growth and neurointegrative development: An experimental ecological study, Pediatrics 38:319, 1966.

33. Kugelmass, I. N., Poull, L. E., and Samuel, E. L. Nutritional improvement of child mentality, Am. J. Med. Sci. 208, 631, 1954.

34. Liang, P. H., Hie, T. T., Jan. O. H., and Glok, L. T. Evaluation of mental development in relation to early malnutrition, Am. J. Clin. Nutr. 20: 1290, 1967.

35. Champakam, S., Srikantia, S. G., and Gopalan, C. Kwashiorkor and mental development, Am. J. Clin. Nutr. 21:844, 1968.

36. Bhatia, C. M. Cited in Performance Tests of Intelligence, London, Oxford University Press, 1958.

37. Hertzig, M. E., Birch, H. G., Richardson, S. A., and Tizard, J. Intellectual levels of school children severely malnourished during the first two years of life, Pediatrics 49:814, 1972.

38. Cravioto, J., Espinoza, C. G., and Birch, H. G. Early malnutrition and auditory-visual integration in school age children, J. Special Education 2:75, 1967.

39. Latham, M. C. Cited in Malnutrition, Learning and Behavior, Scrimshaw, N. S., ed., Cambridge, Mass., M.I.T. Press, 1968, p. 300.

40. Stein, Z., Susser, M., Saenger, G., and Marolla, F., Nutrition and mental performance, Science 178:708, 1972.

41. Lloyd-Still, J. D., Wolff, P. H., Horwitz, I., and Shwachman, H. Studies on intellectual development after severe malnutrition in infancy in cystic fibrosis and other intestinal lesions, Presented at IX International Congress of Nutrition, Mexico, 1972.

42. Klein, R. Personal communication.

43. Campbell, D. T., and Stanley, J. Cited in Experimental and Quasi-Experimental Design for Research, Chicago, Rand McNally & Co., 1969.

44. Schaeffer, E. S. Infant education research project: Implementation and implication of a home tutoring program, in The Pre-School in Action: Exploring Early Childhood Programs, Boston, Allyn & Bacon, 1971.

45. Caldwell, B. M. Descriptive evaluation of child development and of development settings, Pediatrics 40:46, 1967.

46. Skiels, H. M. Adult status of children with contrasting early life experiences, The Society for Research in Child Development, Child Development Monograph Series 31:3, 1966.

47. Winick, M., Meyer, K., and Harris, R. Malnutrition and environmental enrichment by early adoption (in press).

48. McKay, H., McKay, A., and Sinisterra, L. Intellectual development of preschool children in programs of stimulation and nutritional supplementation, in Symposia of the Swedish Nutrition Foundation XIII, Early Malnutrition and Mental Development, Cravioto, J., Hambraeus, L., and Vahlquist, B., eds., Uppsala, Almqvist & Wiksell, 1974, p. 226.

49. Canosa, C. Presented to the Pan American Health Organization Advisory Committee Meeting, 1968.

50. Chow, B. Personal communication.

51. Rush, D., Stein, Z., Christakis, G., and Susser, M. The prenatal project: The first 20 months of operation, in Current Concepts in Nutrition, Vol. 2, Nutrition and Fetal Development, Winick, M., ed., New York, John Wiley & Sons, 1974, p. 95.

52. Chavez, A., Martinez, C., and Yaschine, T. The importance of nutrition and stimuli on child mental and social development, in Symposia of the Swedish Nutrition Foundation XII, Early Malnutrition and Mental Development, Cravioto, J., Hambraeus, L., and Vahlquist, B., eds., Uppsala, Almqvist & Wiksell, 1974, p. 211.

INDEX

Abilities, 140
Ability: abstracting, 139
  integrative, 142
  learning, 130, 138
  memory, 139
  perceptual, 138, 139
  verbal, 139
Abnormalities, behavioral, 136
Abstracting ability, 139
Acetal phosphatide, 45
Acetic inositol phosphatide, 47
N-Acetyl-aspartate, 53
Acetylcholinesterase, 43, 44, 68, 134
N-Acetyl neuraminic acid, 45
Achievement, 149
Achievement scores, 149
Activity: exploratory, 131, 136
  locomotor, 131, 135
  spontaneous, 134
Adductor sesamoid, 16
Adenosine triphosphate (ATP), 49, 50
  content, 49
Adolescence, 15
Adolescents, 24
Adrenaline, 103
Adults, interaction with, 152
Adverse stimuli, 134
Advertising of formulas, 19
Age, 138
Alanine, 52, 53, 54
Albumin: serum, 5, 9, 10, 11
  low, 11, 12
  synthesis, 7, 11
Alkaline phosphatase, heat-stable, 115
Alkaline ribonuclease (RNase), *see*
  Ribnouclease, alkaline
Alpha amino isobutyric acid, 101
Amenorrhea, 25
American Indians, 22

Amid linkage, 45
Amino acids, 9, 11, 51, 52, 57, 58, 79,
  80, 81, 89
  availability, 80, 87
  essential, 7
  glucose conversion to, 57
  incorporation, 56
  increased flow of, 80
  pathways, 80
  pool, 52
  pool size, 80
  transport, 40, 51
  utilization, 40, 51
  γ-amino-butyric acid (GABA), 52,
    53, 54
  shunt, 50, 54
  transaminase, 54
γ-amino-butyril-choline, 54
Aminogram, 11
Ammonia, 52
Ammonium ions, 52
Amniotic fluid, 122, 125
Anaerobiosis, 103
Analysis, retrospective, 146
Ancylostomiasis, 13
Anemia, 7, 13, 23
Animals, isolation of, 136
Anorexia, 12
Anorexia nervosa, 112
Anoxic periods, 50
Anterior fissure, 73
Anthropometry, 22
Anthropomorphic data, 22
Anthropomorphic findings, 23
Anthropomorphic measures, 21
Antioch, siege of, 14
Apathetic state, 132
Apathy, 5, 7, 134, 135
Arachidonic acid, 68

Urea concentration, in rat amniotic
fluid, 122
Urea excretion, 8, 122
Urea production, 9
Urea to creatinine ratio, 8
Urinary/plasma ratio, ribonuclease,
122
Urine, 122
excretion of, 131
fetal, 122
maternal, 125
ribonuclease, 122

Vacuoles, large, 101
Valine, 9, 55
Vascular disease, maternal, 26
Vascular insufficiency, 106, 107, 112
Vasodilation, reflex, 106
Ventral root, 76
fibers, 76
Ventral spinothalamic tract, 73
Ventricle: fourth, 42
lateral, 41, 69, 75, 108
third, 42, 75, 108
Verbal ability, 139
Vertical movement, 131
Villi: peripheral, 114
stem, 114
Villous surface area, 113
Vineland Scale of Social Maturity, 144
Virgin female, rat, 135
Visual-haptic test, 139
Visual integration, 141
Visual placing, 133
Vitamin A, 23, 111
deficit, 24
levels, 24
marginal deficiency, 111
Vitamin B_6, 111

Vitamin B_{12}, 23
Vitamin C, 23
Vulnerability, 94

Water, 38, 49
extracellular, 9
piped, 22
purified, 20
Water mazes, 130
Water retention, 10
Water supply, inadequate, 23
Weakness, 12
Weaning, early, 19
Weanling children, 7
Wechsler Intelligence Scale, 144
for children, 138
for adults, 144
Weight, 15, 37, 119
birth, 144, 152
brain, 64, 117
catch up, 149
control during pregnancy, 26
fetal, 101; brain, 116
gain during pregnancy, 30
per cell, 36
placental, 101, 117
reduction, 26
Weight/DNA ratio, 36, 37, 99
White matter, 45, 46, 47, 73
White persons, 24
Wigglesworth technique, 104
Withdrawal from environment, 134
"Wrapping," 47

Zinc deficiency, 111
in human populations, 112
Zymosterol, 45